THE COMPLETE IDIOT'S GUIDE® TO

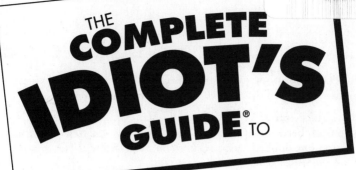

Juicing

by Ellen Brown

ALPHA

A member of Penguin Group (USA) Inc.

ALPHA BOOKS

Published by the Penguin Group

Penguin Group (USA) Inc., 375 Hudson Street, New York, New York 10014, U.S.A.

Penguin Group (Canada), 10 Alcorn Avenue, Toronto, Ontario, Canada M4V 3B2 (a division of Pearson Penguin Canada Inc.)

Penguin Books Ltd, 80 Strand, London WC2R 0RL, England

Penguin Ireland, 25 St Stephen's Green, Dublin 2, Ireland (a division of Penguin Books Ltd)

Penguin Group (Australia), 250 Camberwell Road, Camberwell, Victoria 3124, Australia (a division of Pearson Australia Group Pty Ltd)

Penguin Books India Pvt Ltd, 11 Community Centre, Panchsheel Park, New Delhi—110 017, India

Penguin Group (NZ), cnr Airborne and Rosedale Roads, Albany, Auckland 1310, New Zealand (a division of Pearson New Zealand Ltd)

Penguin Books (South Africa) (Pty) Ltd, 24 Sturdee Avenue, Rosebank, Johannesburg 2196, South Africa

Penguin Books Ltd, Registered Offices: 80 Strand, London WC2R 0RL, England

International Standard Book Number: 978-1-59257-568-8
Library of Congress Catalog Card Number: 2006930729

09   8   7   6   5   4

Interpretation of the printing code: The rightmost number of the first series of numbers is the year of the book's printing; the rightmost number of the second series of numbers is the number of the book's printing. For example, a printing code of 07-1 shows that the first printing occurred in 2007.

Printed in the United States of America

Note: This publication contains the opinions and ideas of its author. It is intended to provide helpful and informative material on the subject matter covered. It is sold with the understanding that the author and publisher are not engaged in rendering professional services in the book. If the reader requires personal assistance or advice, a competent professional should be consulted.

The author and publisher specifically disclaim any responsibility for any liability, loss, or risk, personal or otherwise, which is incurred as a consequence, directly or indirectly, of the use and application of any of the contents of this book.

Most Alpha books are available at special quantity discounts for bulk purchases for sales promotions, premiums, fund-raising, or educational use. Special books, or book excerpts, can also be created to fit specific needs.

For details, write: Special Markets, Alpha Books, 375 Hudson Street, New York, NY 10014.

Publisher: *Marie Butler-Knight*
Editorial Director: *Mike Sanders*
Managing Editor: *Billy Fields*
Acquisitions Editor: *Michele Wells*
Development Editor: *Nancy D. Lewis*
Senior Production Editor: *Janette Lynn*
Copy Editor: *Nancy Wagner*
Cover/Book Designers: *Kurt Owens/Trina Wurst*
Indexer: *Brad Herriman*
Layout: *Ayanna Lacey*
Proofreader: *John Etchison*

Contents at a Glance

Contents

Appendixes

Introduction

There's nothing new about juicing. We've given it a snappy handle, but juicing's been around for centuries. Drinking the juices of raw fruits and vegetables as a path to good health was even touted in the early nineteenth century.

While juicing itself isn't new, what *is* new is the machine that can render even the hardest beet into a sweet juice to sip in a matter of seconds. This ability is increasingly important as our society quantifies the amounts of these foods we should be eating. Some governmental agencies say five daily servings of vegetables and three of fruit, while other medical groups advocate seven vegetables and two fruits. Regardless of exact number, it's a lot.

That's where the benefits of juicing begin. An 8-ounce glass of juice can fulfill a third of your daily needs. It's like the difference in medicine between injections and pills. The benefits of the injection go directly into your bloodstream, while a pill must dissolve and be absorbed, which increases the time between when you take it and when you begin to feel the results.

The same is true when juicing because it allows the body to quickly absorb high-quality nutrition, which leads to increased energy levels. So drinking fresh juices is an excellent health habit. It's more than an excellent source of vitamins, minerals, enzymes, purified water, proteins, carbohydrates, and chlorophyll. In liquid form, juices supply nutrition that is not wasted on creating its own digestion, as is the case when eating whole fruits or juices with a large percentage of pulp.

Here are some of the benefits that come from juicing:

◆ **Juicing creates fast assimilation of nutrients.** Some enzymes, vitamins, and minerals are "trapped" in the indigestible fiber of vegetables and fruits and can take up to a few hours to be assimilated into the body. When these nutrients are added as a pure juice, the time is reduced to 15 minutes, which allows the body to rest.

◆ **Juicing keeps up our water table.** Our cells consist mostly of water, which is essential to their proper function. That's why we should consume at least 8 glasses of water a day. Beverages such as coffee, soft drinks, and alcohol actually draw water from our bodies to metabolize. Raw juices, on the other hand, supply the water we need to replenish lost fluid. And the water is purified better than from any bottle. Juices also promote our bodies' natural alkalinity, which is important for immune systems and metabolic functions to work properly.

◆ **Juices deliver natural sugar.** The natural sugars in fruits and vegetables deliver the same energy as from soft drinks but without chemicals or fat.

You might be wondering why I'm asking you to buy an expensive machine rather than just pour from a bottle. There's an important reason: only fresh juices that haven't been pasteurized to increase their stability contain necessary enzymes and other "living" ingredients.

Plants are the spark plugs that keep our bodies running. They get their energy from the sun during photosynthesis. These "living" qualities comprise enzymes, vitamins, and minerals. Minerals are basic parts of the earth's crust, and plants get them from the soil while enzymes and vitamins are produced in plants' tissues.

But cooking and processing destroy these nutrients. Enter juicing as a way to get the maximum benefit. Cooking accounts for the loss of almost all the water-soluble vitamins (A, E, D, and K) from food. And even allowing raw vegetables to sit after peeling reduces their level of nutrients. For example, cantaloupes lose 35 percent of their vitamin C if slices sit overnight in the refrigerator.

So drinking a juice right after it's extracted gives you the best of all possible worlds.

How This Book Is Organized

The book is divided into four parts:

Part 1, "Component Parts," teaches you the fundamentals of juicing. The first chapter details how to select a juicer, how to use your blender, and the difference between juicing and pulping. In the next two chapters you'll find profiles of fruits and vegetables frequently specified in recipes, along with their nutritional highlights and the amount of juice that comes from them. Part 1 ends with a chapter detailing information on nutritional supplements you can add to juices, herbs you can use to flavor them, and ways to use your juice machine as a kitchen tool.

Part 2, "Garden Patch Purées," gives you combinations that use just about all the vegetables in the produce aisle. The recipes are divided by both the types of vegetables they contain and if any additional ingredients are added into the flavor profile. In one chapter juices are made primarily from root vegetables, and the next showcases the cabbage and its cousins. The rest of the chapters in Part 2 are for juices complexly flavored with herbs, based on popular cold soups, or balancing fruits with the vegetables.

Part 3, "Fruity and Fantastic," shows you that often the whole is better than the sum of its parts. Juice is almost synonymous with fruit, and these recipes multiply the ways you can combine these luscious juices. The recipes in Part 3 are divided by the nature of the predominant fruit in the juice blend. They range from tropical treats to bowls full of bright berries.

Part 4, "Lean and Luscious Libations," demonstrates that juices can be fun as well as serious. These juices are meant for parties, either as punches or as cocktails. The recipes in the first chapter of Part 4 are all flavored teas. Some use herbal teas while others encompass many species of prized black tea. In the last chapter of Part 4, you'll see some sort of alcohol listed amongst the ingredients, but instructions are given on how to concoct the juices to remain "unleaded."

At the end you'll find some useful appendixes. A glossary will add to your knowledge of foods, and an appendix of charts will help you convert measurements to the metric system. The last appendix is a chart listing the nutritional composition of the fruits and vegetables frequently used in these recipes.

Extras

In every chapter you'll find boxes that give you extra information that is either helpful, interesting, or both.

Juicy Jive

Juicy Jive boxes are where you'll find tips. Some are specific to the recipes they accompany; others will boost your general knowledge of juicing and its ingredients or give you ideas for presentation. These tips are meant to make your life easier and your time in the kitchen more pleasurable.

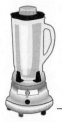

Pulp Tidbits

Check out these boxes for amusing tidbits of food history. They're fun to read and share with friends, and they'll make you sound like a real gourmet.

Wrong Spin!

It's always a good idea to be alerted to potential problems in advance. Boxes labeled Wrong Spin! provide just such warnings, either about cooking in general or the recipe in particular.

Liquid Lingo

All cooking—including juicing—has a language all its own, and some of the terms and ingredients can be intimidating if you don't know what they mean. Look to these boxes for technique and ingredient definitions if you don't want to flip to the glossary.

Nutritional Analysis

All the recipes in this book have been annotated with some nutritional information so you know what you're drinking. Because these recipes are meant as food and not as medicine, the analysis does not detail every mineral or vitamin. It does provide you with some useful information so you know what nutrients you're gaining from the juice.

Acknowledgments

Writing a book is a solitary endeavor, but its publication is always a team effort. My thanks go to …

Michele Wells of Alpha Books and Ed Claflin, my agent, for proposing the project.

Nancy Lewis and Nancy Wagner for their expert and eagle-eyed editing.

Tigger–Cat Brown and Patches–Kitten Brown, my furry companions, who kept me company for endless hours at the computer.

Special Thanks to the Technical Reviewer

The Complete Idiot's Guide to Juicing was reviewed by an expert who provided the nutritional analysis of each recipe, to help us ensure that this book gives you everything you need to know about juicing. Special thanks are extended to Karen Konopelski, R.D.

Karen is a Registered Dietitian and is currently pursing a Master's degree in Nutrition with a concentration in Exercise and Sports at the University of Connecticut. She also develops diet plans and counsels collegiate and professional athletes to maximize performance.

Trademarks

Part 1

Component Parts

If you can use a knife, you can make any juice in this book. Not only do you need no culinary skills or a stove, but you don't even need to have teeth.

These chapters contain all the information you'll need to start juicing! First I discuss the necessary machines, and then I give you chapters on fruits and vegetables to put through the juicer.

Juicing is like jazz. Once you have a classical foundation, you can begin to improvise, so this part ends with a chapter that presents other ingredients you might want to add to juices.

Just Juicing

In This Chapter

- Juicing is smart
- The pulping alternative
- Types of juicers
- The importance of organics

You already know that it's smart to add fresh juices to your diet. That's why you're holding this book. Right? So now let me validate your hunch with solid information.

Nutritional Necessities

Every health organization—including the American Cancer Society, the National Cancer Institute, and the National Research Council—believes Americans don't eat enough fresh fruits and vegetables to prevent disease.

And cooking and processing destroys food's natural *nutrients* and energy, so you're not getting as many benefits from eating the food if you cook it. But juicing preserves all those nutrients.

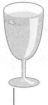

Liquid Lingo

Nutrients are elements or compounds that our bodies need for metabolism, growth, or other functioning. Carbohydrates, proteins, and fats are the three substances that provide energy in our diets, while vitamins, minerals, and water are the essential nutrients that support metabolism. All of these come from the foods we eat.

Vitamins for Vitality

To remain healthy, humans need to consume some 13 vitamins a day. The largest group of these vitamins is the eight distinct B vitamins and also vitamin C, which are all water soluble. This means that with the exception of vitamin B12, which is stored in the liver, you need to eat foods that contain these vitamins on a daily basis because they don't stick around. You know many of these vitamins in the B family by their chemical names, such as thiamine (B1), niacin (B3), and folic acid (B9).

Pulp Tidbits

Casimar Funk, a Polish chemist in the early 1900s, set out to research diseases like rickets and scurvy. He discovered that these widespread maladies were due to chemical deficiencies rather than poisons in the diet. He named these chemical compounds *vitamins*, or literally "union of vitality."

The body stores the fat-soluble vitamins, which is both good and bad. On the good side, you can go for a day or so without meeting your quota and your body will still function well. But on the bad side, too much of a fat-soluble vitamin can lead to toxicity.

Magic from Minerals

Dietary minerals are the group of nutrients that bind us to all living organisms. Plants need them to prosper and grow and so do humans. The mineral content of food depends on the soil in which it's planted. Soil is the natural breakdown of the minerals in the rocks that form the earth, and some soils are richer in some minerals than others.

The trace minerals include chromium, cobalt, copper, fluorine, iodine, iron, and magnesium. Of these, the body needs iodine in the largest quantity, which is why table salt frequently has iodine added as a dietary supplement.

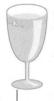

Liquid Lingo

Dietary minerals are the chemical elements required by all living organisms. They can either be bulk minerals our bodies require in large amounts or trace minerals that we only need a small amount of in our diets to keep us healthy.

Essential Enzymes

Enzymes are the body's worker bees because they are constantly demolishing and rebuilding our bodies. Approximately 1,000 enzymes are found in all living things, including raw food. It's the enzymes in fruits and vegetables that cause them to ripen.

Juicy Jive

Enzymes are paired with the foods they help to break down. For example, bananas are high in carbohydrates and contain amylase which is a carbohydrate-splitting enzyme. Butter is high in saturated fat and contains lipase, an enzyme that splits fat.

Amino Acids

Next to water, protein is the most plentiful element in the body, and more than 50 percent of the dry weight of the body is composed of protein. Proteins, in turn, are composed of protein chains called amino acids. These amino acids are the raw materials with which the enzymes do their building.

The essential amino acids are those that the body can gain only from the foods we eat. A deficiency in an amino acid can create a range of symptoms from allergies to poor digestion. For example:

◆ Lysine helps to activate hormones and enzymes, as well as promote body growth and blood circulation.

- Leucine keeps us awake and alert. It's sort of nature's own jolt of caffeine.

- Tryptophan is essential for building blood, skin, and hair. It also calms the nerves and stimulates digestion.

- Phenylalanine is what gives the thyroid gland a boost in the production of thyroxin for our mental balance.

- Threonine stimulates easy digestion and general body metabolism.

- Valine activates the brain, helps in muscle coordination, and calms the nerves.

- Methionine helps cleanse both the liver and kidneys and regenerate their cells.

Pulp Tidbits

Did you ever wonder why you're always so mellow after Thanksgiving dinner? Sure, you ate a lot of food. But one of those foods was turkey, which contains a high amount of tryptophan. So after your turkey dinner, you're calm—and full.

The need for nutrients and increasing their number in your diet is the "why" of juicing. Now it's time to get to the "how" of juicing.

Passion for Pulping

Let's say you don't want to invest in a juicer when you already have a blender and perhaps a food processor. Well, don't despair. You can still gain lots of beneficial food energy with a process called pulping. This process works the same as juicing, but if you want to drink the mixture without the pulp, you will need to strain the resulting liquid.

Fundamentals of Fiber

Vegetables and fruits are full of two different types of fiber, and fiber is necessary in the diet. That's why if you're using a juicer, you have to remain aware of how much fiber you've had in the course of a day from other sources, such as whole grains, nuts, and seeds.

The first type is insoluble fiber. Water does nothing to its size or form, but it helps to keep stools soft in the intestinal tract and push them through the tract faster. This is the type of fiber found in whole wheat, wheat and corn bran, and potato skins.

Then there's the soluble fiber. Soluble fiber forms a soft gel when it mixes with water in our bodies and is able to bind bile salts which may help in lowering cholesterol. It also keeps the digestive tract functioning properly. When a drink is pulped, this beneficial fiber is retained with all the good things from the juice.

Pulp Tidbits

Eating large quantities of beans and other legumes can cause potentially embarrassing bouts of gas and other forms of flatulence because they contain short-chain carbohydrates that are not digested by the human digestive tract but by natural bacteria in the colon. It's just nature doing its thing.

Prepping Your Parts

It would be easy if all you had to do was place the produce in the blender to pulp it. But it's not that easy. Blenders and food processors don't separate the juice from the pulp. They create a thick liquefied mixture by puréeing. So for each recipe, I give you tips on how to prepare the food for pulping as well as juicing.

In a juicer the tops of scallions will be ejected along with all the other pulp. But for a blender or food processor, you should cut off the tops for aesthetic reasons. The same holds true for the skin of yams and some fruit skins.

Wrong Spin!

If you want to peel apples, pears, or bananas for pulping, either do so just before blending them or else toss them with some fresh lemon juice to prevent them from browning. While the browning does not change the flavor, it gives these fruits a most unappealing color.

Machines with Muscle

When you're thinking about a juicer, don't picture that little plastic thing you use to squeeze lemon juice. That's about as close to a real juicer as the Wright brothers' airplane is to the Space Shuttle. The juicers we're discussing are powerful machines. They have to be. Their purpose is to separate the liquid from the fiber, and that takes power. Consider how hard it would be to squeeze the juice from a beet using the little plastic thing you use for lemons.

Choosing Your Weapon

When selecting a juicer, it's most important to choose one with a stable motor and low heat generation. Excess heat will instantly kill out enzymes. The stability of the machine as it's doing its appointed task is more important than the number of rpms (revolutions per minute) it boasts. The more efficiently the unit can shred and eject pulp, the less the possibility that the juicer will clog or overheat.

Juicers fall into the following categories:

◆ **Masticating:** Food is squeezed through gears that crush it and force it through a fine strainer. Pulp is continuously extracted, and nutrients are preserved because the machine doesn't generate heat or friction.

> **Juicy Jive**
>
> Few stores will allow you to try juicers before purchasing them, but that's where the Internet enters the picture. Take down the names of juicers that interest you, and check out the manufacturers' websites. Chances are you'll find a video demonstration, which is the next best thing to personally testing the machine.

◆ **Centrifugal:** A spinning basket shreds the food and forces the juice through a fine strainer by centrifugal force. This process adds oxygen to the juices and makes them somewhat frothy.

Either type works efficiently and is up to the task at hand. You'll find information on how it functions on the box.

Preventing Buyer's Remorse

At most department and discount stores, you'll see a wall of juicers displayed, which makes it difficult to select one. They'll range in price from about $75 to more than $350. I'm sorry to tell you that powerful motors aren't cheap.

Consider these guidelines when selecting a juicer:

◆ Is it easy to use and clean? In general, I find centrifugal juices are easier to handle than their masticating cousins.

◆ What is the percentage of juice it removes from the pulp? It should be at least 90 percent.

◆ How much juice will it process before you have to empty the container and the pulp container? If the juice beaker only holds a cup, it slows down the process.

◆ Does it have different speeds for different jobs? Most of the good ones have high and low, with high used for harder foods.

◆ Does it sit securely on the counter? This is a major consideration, as well as whether the feed tube is easy to use at your height.

◆ How noisy is it? Some juicers I tried require earplugs to save your hearing, while others are virtually silent. In general the centrifugal juicers are quieter, as are juicers that are more expensive.

◆ Can the parts go into the dishwasher? To me this is a deal breaker. I don't want any machine that can't go into my favorite machine.

Before rushing out with credit card in hand, spend some time researching your options online. Many companies will give user reviews, and cyber shopping is also a way to find a good deal!

> **Juicy Jive**
>
> Don't throw away the pulp from the juicer if you're a gardener or even know one. It makes rich compost to add into soil once it has broken down, but don't just put it on top of your flower beds or you'll be inviting a bug invasion. You can also add the pulp to soups as a thickening agent.

Completing the Equipment List

No machine exists in a vacuum. So here's a list of smaller items you'll need to join into juicing:

- A selection of sharp knives for peeling and coring
- A stiff brush for scrubbing vegetables like carrots
- A peeler that removes the thinnest amount of skin possible
- Plastic cutting boards
- A sieve for straining
- Measuring cups and measuring spoons
- Flexible rubber spatulas

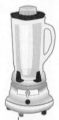

Wrong Spin!

Cutting boards, along with sponges, are the petri dishes of a kitchen. Those pretty wooden ones allow bacteria to grow. The best cutting boards are heavy plastic that can go into the dishwasher every time you use them.

Blender Basics

Chances are you already own a blender, and if you do, then you're all set both for pulping and for incorporating foods as a second step to juicing.

Many recipes in this book specify the use of a blender or food processor as well as a juicer. The primary reason is that foods such as bananas and avocadoes don't contain enough water to juice correctly. You would end up with virtually no juice or nutrients. The second reason is that certain foods such as seasonings don't juice well, so you're instructed to either add them via a blender or stir them into the juices by hand.

Purchase Prowess

If you're buying a new blender, you don't have to mortgage the house. When blender shopping, look for a blender that has …

◆ A heavy base to stabilize it on the counter.

◆ A strong motor of 60 hertz or more. This makes it strong enough to chop the hardest vegetable, and it will last far longer than machines with less power.

◆ A glass jar so that it's dishwasher safe. Some of the most expensive blenders have stainless-steel jars. They are the most durable, yes, but you can't see what's going on inside.

◆ A two-piece lid that fits very snugly on the jar to avoid leaks. The small access hole in the center of the lid allows you to add ingredients when the machine is running.

> **Juicy Jive**
>
> When you're blender shopping, consider how easy or inexpensive it would be to replace the jar or purchase a second jar. This could make the difference between two machines at a similar price point.

Operating Instructions

A blender might look innocuous enough, but you definitely need to approach this machine with caution. These usage tips will help you get the most from your blender:

◆ Always keep one hand on the top of the lid to ensure it won't fly off.

◆ Turn off the blender completely and allow the liquid to stop moving before removing the lid.

◆ Never put your hands in the blender jar, and be sure the blades have stopped moving before you insert a spatula into the jar.

◆ Use only rubber spatulas, not metal spoons or knives.

◆ Never fill a blender more than two-thirds full. When the motor moves the liquid around, it will push it above the level of the ingredients at rest. Never fill it too full, or you could have a mess.

The Organic Alternative

Whenever you have the chance, it's always best to buy produce that is certified organic. Organic agriculture is about growing foods without synthetic fertilizers and chemical biocides. And it's also about using agricultural practices that benefit the planet, such as recycling.

Each year more than a billion pounds of pesticides and herbicides are used in the United States. About 2 percent actually kill insects, with the remaining 98 percent ending up in the air, water, soil, and food supply. But this is not the case with organic foods.

When this method of healthy farming began about 20 years ago, the only way to ensure that food was organic was to purchase it directly from a reputable farmer. Luckily, that's no longer the case.

In 2002 the National Organic Program (NOP) became law. The U.S. Department of Agriculture administers this program, which upholds the prohibitions against chemicals first spelled out in the Organic Food Production Act of 1990. The NOP states that it believes in "optimizing the health and productivity of interdependent communities of soil life, plants, animals, and people. Management practices are carefully selected with an intent to restore and then maintain ecological harmony on the farm, its surrounding environment, and ultimately the whole planetary ecosystem."

Wanting to eat organic food is another reason to buy food in season rather than imported. While many European countries also

Juicy Jive

Make buying organic your shopping goal when you're looking for shelf-stable food as well as fresh. There are now organic options for everything from canned tomatoes and chicken stock to tortilla chips made from organic corn. These are all good choices.

have strict standards as to the meaning of "organic," the same cannot be said for most Asian and Latin American countries—and they are the source of most crops that are out of season in the United States.

When using produce that is conventional rather than organic, always pay attention to the skin to see if it's been treated with wax. This is especially true of cucumbers and citrus fruits. While citrus fruits need to be peeled before juicing, cucumbers do not. But if they are waxed, it is necessary to peel them.

The Least You Need to Know

◆ Juicing is an effective way of delivering nutrients to our bodies.

◆ Pulping uses the same ingredients as juicing but leaves in the fiber because pulped drinks are made in a blender.

◆ Juicers remove the juice from the pulp either by centrifugal force or through mastication.

◆ Organic produce is the best to use at all times because it's not subjected to chemicals.

Chapter 2

Fruits for All Seasons

In This Chapter

- ◆ Fruits to juice
- ◆ Juice yields
- ◆ Tips for freezing fruit

Fruit and juice are synonymous to most people. If you only drink one glass of juice a day, chances are it's a fruit juice in the morning. In this chapter, I'll give you a guide to the fruits that I most often use in the recipes in this book. You'll learn how to tell if fruits are ripe and ready for juicing and how to freeze ripe fruit for future treats.

You'll also get some handy knowledge about how much juice you'll get from various fruits. This is useful if you're using juices for these recipes that someone else has squeezed.

Nature's Energy

Fruits contain both complex carbohydrates and simple sugars. The complex carbohydrates are more slowly digested, which keeps your energy level up.

The simple sugars are in a form called fructose. In contrast to complex carbohydrates, fructose gives you instant energy when you drink the juice, but it also gives you nutrients you won't get from the "empty calories" from refined sugar.

The Fruit Family

What unites fruit botanically as a group is that it has a seed or many seeds. That's why tomatoes, eggplant, and avocadoes are technically fruits. But because we eat them as vegetables and with other vegetables, we'll discuss them in Chapter 3.

The majority of this chapter gives you profiles of different fruits. At the end of the discussion of some fruits, I tell you how much juice you might expect to extract. So if you want to use a high-quality bottled juice, you'll know the equivalents.

Apples. Although not as high in vitamins as some other fruits, apples do contain a high level of pectin, which helps reduce cholesterol. Yield: 8 ounces of juice per pound of apples.

Apricots. High in beta-carotene, which the body converts to vitamin A, pale ripe apricots are also a good source of fiber and potassium. A ripe apricot is soft when gently pressed, and the skin is thin enough that it does not have to be peeled. Just slice the apricot and discard the pit. Yield: 6 ounces of juice per pound of apricots.

Bananas. Bananas are an easy way to get a juice with a creamy texture without adding cream—or any binder for that matter. They are a fantastic source of potassium, an electrolyte lost during exercise, as well as an excellent source of magnesium and vitamin B6. Bananas are truly ripe when the peels are mottled with brown spots, not just bright yellow. Yield: 2 ounces of juice per pound of bananas.

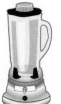

Wrong Spin!

Bananas should not be pushed through your juicer. Because they don't contain very much juice, you won't have the luscious texture they bring to juices when they're added in a blender.

Blackberries. Blackberries, rich, purple-black in color and high in heart-healthy compounds called saponins, are actually a cluster of tiny fruits, each with its own seed. They're most common and affordable during the summer and can be successfully frozen after a quick rinse and gentle patting with paper towels. Yield: 4 ounces of juice per pound of blackberries.

Blueberries. In addition to antioxidant vitamins, blueberries are high in salicylate, a compound that reduces inflammation. Look for berries that are plump, not shriveled, and have a slight grayish patina. Rinse them, discard any stems, twigs, or small green berries, and they're ready to go. You can use blueberries fresh, or dry them on paper towels and freeze them in a plastic bag. Yield: 3 ounces of juice per pound of blueberries.

Cantaloupes. Cantaloupes are rich in beta-carotene, vitamin C, and potassium. The rind should appear well netted. To tell if it was picked ripe, look at the stem end. It should be a full scar, without flesh attached, showing that it was picked when mature. Cantaloupe can be a carrier of salmonella, so wash the rind with soap and water before peeling it. Yield: 8 ounces of juice per pound of cantaloupe.

Cranberries. It's not a wives' tale: cranberries, high in vitamin C, do alleviate bladder infections because they prevent bacteria from attaching to the wall of the bladder. Select plump, non-shriveled cranberries and rinse them in a colander. It's difficult to find fresh cranberries except in the fall, so buy a few extra bags when you can find them, and freeze them for use during the year by rinsing them and placing them in plastic bags. Yield: 4 ounces of juice per pound of cranberries.

Wrong Spin!

Because it can be quite acidic, most bottled cranberry juice is either sweetened with corn syrup or other sweeteners or blended with apple or grape juices (often with less cranberry than the other juice). If you want real cranberry flavor, look for smaller brands and in health food stores to find the real thing.

Cherries. Rich in potassium and B vitamins, sweet cherries come in a range of colors and all make great juices. Discard the stems, rinse the cherries in a colander, cut them in half and discard the pits, and they're ready to go. Yield: 6 to 8 ounces per pound of cherries.

Grapes. Both green and red grapes are high in potassium, and their flavor is almost identical. Which one you choose depends on your aesthetic preference and which seems the sweetest. Rinse and remove grapes from the stems; then dry on paper towels. Yield: 8 ounces per pound of grapes.

Pulp Tidbits

There are approximately 8,000 varieties of grapes, many of which date back to prehistoric times. The main classifications we now follow are the difference between wine grapes, which are high in acid, and table grapes, which are sweet. Thomas Jefferson was the first person to try to raise wine grapes in the United States.

Juicy Jive

Melons are the juiciest of fruits, and some of the juice can be lost when you're peeling them. Always handle melons over a mixing bowl to catch the sweet juice. Then strain the juice and toss it into the beaker with the juice coming out of your machine.

Honeydews. A good source of both potassium and vitamin C, choose honeydews that are green, not white, and slightly perfumed. Cut honeydew melons into quarters, and then cut away the soft flesh from the hard peel. Since the fruit is being pushed through a juicer, how pretty it looks is irrelevant. Yield: 6 ounces of juice per pound of honeydew melon.

Kiwi. Kiwi are a rich source of vitamin C, and their potassium level is almost as high as that of bananas. They contain both vitamin A and E, and their fuzzy skin can be used as a meat tenderizer in the same way as papaya skin. When juicing, it's not necessary to peel the kiwi, and the skin contains some valuable antioxidants. But when pulping, do peel them. Yield: 4 ounces of juice per pound of kiwi.

Mangoes. Like other orange-fleshed fruits, mangoes are a good choice for beta-carotene. Mangoes are ripe if they're slightly soft when pressed and the skin is mottled with red and orange. Avoid buying rock-hard green mangoes because they might never ripen. Yield: 5 ounces of juice per pound of mangoes.

Juicy Jive

Mangoes have a hard way and an easy way of being peeled, which varies fruit to fruit. If you're having problems cutting away the skin, try peeling it from the other end. The stone (pit) is elliptical, and once you've determined its shape, cut a parallel slit on both sides to remove as much flesh as possible; then cut off any flesh remaining on the stone.

Nectarines. See Peaches.

Oranges. Oranges are a superb source of vitamin C. For juicing, it's only necessary to peel an orange. The white pith will be ejected with the other pulp. When placing them in a blender, the best way to prepare oranges is to cut off the top and bottom so the orange will sit snugly on the work surface. Then use a serrated fruit knife to cut off the peel, including the white pith. Cut between the white lines that mark the sections, and the orange sections, sans peel, will pop right out. Yield: 8 ounces of juice per pound of oranges.

Papayas. Nutritionally, the papaya is best known as a source of the enzyme *papain*. Buy papayas somewhat soft and golden orange. If the fruit is hard, cut a small slice off both ends, then make a few lengthwise cuts into the flesh. The papaya will ripen in a few days at room temperature. Always peel the papaya and discard the peppery seeds before cubing it. Yield: 1 to 3 ounces of juice per pound of papaya.

Liquid Lingo

Papain is an enzyme that can ease indigestion and has been shown to protect the stomach from ulcers. It is also a tenderizer, so save papaya skins and toss them into a meat marinade to speed along tenderizing meats.

Peaches. Peaches, high in beta-carotene, are ripe if they're soft when pressed gently. There's no reason to peel peaches before pushing them through the juicer; however, you might want to peel them if

Juicy Jive

There are two basic types of peaches, cling-stone and freestone. They taste similar, and the only difference is whether or not the flesh clings to the pit. Both make an excellent juice, and regard-less of which you pick, choose the ripest peach you can find.

they're destined for the blender. If so, drop them into boiling water for 30 seconds, remove and drain lightly, and the skins will slip right off when you rub the fruit. Yield: 1 to 3 ounces of juice per pound of peaches.

Pears. Fiber-rich pears are a good source of vitamin C and potassium. Pears ripen better off the tree, and it might take up to a week for them to ripen if they're rock-hard when you buy them. You can substitute any variety of pear for another. Yield: 4 to 6 ounces of juice per pound of pears.

Pineapples. Pineapples are a good source of minerals, including potassium, calcium, iron, and iodine. Choose one that is fragrant and plump with an overall golden color, or allow it to sit at room tempera-ture until it meets that description. Slice off the top and bottom so it sits flat on your work surface. Then, with a strong knife, slice off the peel. It's not necessary to remove the tough core when juicing or pulp-ing pineapples. Yield: 6 ounces of juice per pound of pineapple.

Juicy Jive

Plums have a crease on one side that runs paral-lel to the flat side of the pit. Slice plums lengthwise along the crease, and you should be able to see the pit. Discard it, and you're ready to slice or dice.

Plums. Rich in antioxidant vitamin C, all the hundreds of species of plums are good in juices if they're ripe. A plum is ripe if it's soft when you gently press it with your finger. Just rinse plums before slicing them, and discard the pit. Peeling is not necessary. Yield: 4 ounces of juice per pound of plums.

Raspberries. Vitamin C is the big boast of succulent raspberries, which are now grown in a rainbow of colors, from classic red to golden amber. When choosing fresh raspberries, look at the bottom of the container, and choose one that has the least amount of juice, a sign that the berries are not damaged or moldy. Place berries in a bowl of water, stir them around to dislodge any lingering dirt, and then gently pat them dry on paper towels. Yield: 4 to 5 ounces of juice per pound of raspberries.

Strawberries. A good source of iron as well as B vitamins and vitamin C, strawberries do not ripen once they've been picked, so what you buy is what you get. Because most companies "top dress" the packages with the "hero berries" on the top, check out the bottom of the package. Generally, the smaller the berry, the more intense the flavor. Tiny European *fraises du bois* are the sweetest of all. Yield: 4 to 5 ounces of juice per pound of strawberries.

Pulp Tidbits

Raspberries were a campaign issue in a presidential election. Because they were considered quite the luxury, in 1840 the Whigs attacked Martin Van Buren for "wallowing lasciviously in raspberries."

Liquid Lingo

Fraises du bois literally means "strawberries of the woods" in French, and you can find these tiny treats in specialty produce markets, most often in the spring. Treat them as you would any other berry.

Watermelons. Watermelon is rich in electrolytes, which makes it a good choice for a snack after a strenuous workout or any other time you might be dehydrated. One of the great feats of genetic engineering is the seedless watermelon. They're not as much fun because you can't spit the seeds at your friends, but they're much easier to transform into a juice. It's easier to cut the flesh off the rind after cutting a watermelon in quarters than it is to cut through the rock-hard rind. It's not necessary to remove the seeds when juicing, but it is important if pulping watermelon. The best idea is

Juicy Jive

Watermelon doesn't produce more juice because the rind is so dense and heavy. Per ounce of edible flesh, watermelon is one of the highest juice producers.

to buy seedless ones. Yield: 6 to 8 ounces of juice per pound of watermelon.

Supporting Players

Lemons and limes, both rich in vitamin C, are never used in large quantities in juices due to their lip-pursing tartness. But in small quantities their tartness creates a yin-yang with sweeter fruits and accentuates the other fruits' flavors.

When choosing lemons and limes, look for ones with thin skins because they'll have more juice. The yield for both fruit is 4 ounces of juice per pound.

Fresh from the Freezer

Modern air transportation has given us a new definition of "airline food," and we can now enjoy almost all fruits year-round thanks to air freight from other countries. But we do pay a price for this convenience, so for juicing, it's also possible to take advantage of *dry-packed frozen fruits*.

If you stock up on fruits when they are either in season locally or attractively priced and then freeze them yourself, you'll save money plus have a freezer stocked. Do keep in mind that you lose some of the nutrients when fruit is frozen, but many remain intact.

Liquid Lingo

Dry-packed frozen fruits are frozen in individual pieces without any syrup or additional sugar. You'll find the fruits in plastic bags in the freezer section of your supermarket.

The best way to freeze fruit is to first prepare the fruit by cleaning, slicing, peeling, sectioning, etc. as appropriate. Then simply arrange ½- to 1-inch pieces on a baking sheet, cover with plastic wrap, and put them into the freezer until they're frozen. Once frozen, transfer the fruit to a heavy, resealable plastic bag. Mark the date on the bag, and use the fruit within two months.

The Least You Need to Know

- ◆ Fruits contain both complex carbohydrates and simple sugars.
- ◆ It is not necessary to peel apples, peaches, or pears prior to juicing them.
- ◆ Papaya skin contains an enzyme that tenderizes meats, so save it for marinades.
- ◆ Dry-packed frozen foods are preferable to fruits packed in sugar syrup.

3

Versatile Veggies

In This Chapter

- ◆ Vegetables to juice
- ◆ Picking the best produce
- ◆ Juice yields

I grew up knowing vegetables were turned into juice. After all, restaurants served tomato juice as an hors d'oeuvre, and then V-8 made a splash and declared it contained eight vegetables, although I doubt I could name them all. Then I discovered gazpacho as a cooling summer soup. That was just one step away from a mixed vegetable juice.

We've come a long way, and we now appreciate how nutrient-rich vegetable juices can add to our general health. In this chapter I give listings of vegetables that are frequently juiced. Each contains the nutritional highlights of the vegetable, along with how to select it and store it.

Successful Shopping

Shopping for vegetables is much easier than shopping for fruit. Vegetables don't need to ripen to gain greatness. In fact, it's just the opposite. Vegetables should be eaten as soon as possible after they're picked.

In an ideal world, we'd pick vegetables from the garden outside the kitchen door and enjoy them within minutes. But we know that's a bit unrealistic and probably wouldn't offer enough variety.

Juicy Jive

Always rinse all produce just before juicing it or cooking it. Water can cause any leafy vegetable or herb to rot or mold more quickly than if it's stored dry.

It's best to buy vegetables at least two or three times a week, and always try to use up what's in the refrigerator before replenishing them. In the listings I talk about how long vegetables can be stored, but especially with organic vegetables that are not subjected to waxing and other forms of preservation, it's always best to deplete your supply quickly.

From Asparagus to Zucchini

Unlike fruits, vegetables have no common denominator other than they somehow came from the earth. Some grow above ground, while others grow below.

Here's a guide to vegetables frequently pushed through the juicer:

Asparagus. Asparagus, a good source of vitamins A and B1 as well as folic acid, is actually a member of the lily family. The young shoot is the edible part, and while most of our asparagus is green, it can also be white or purple. When choosing asparagus, look for straight firm stalks with tightly closed buds. The stem end should still be firm because it dries out as it ages. In the early spring, buy very thin asparagus, but the fatter stalks will have more flavor in May and June. Asparagus begins to lose flavor as soon as it is picked, but it can be stored up to three days. Wrap the stems in a damp paper towel. For juicing, all you have to do is rinse the spears and cut them into 2-inch lengths, but for cooking it's generally desirable to break off the woody stems and peel the bottom few inches of the stalks. Yield: 6 ounces of juice per pound of asparagus.

Avocado. Avocado is a great source of potassium, and is also high in vitamins A, C, and E. These buttery members of the pear family are so perishable that they're always shipped to stores when rock hard. Look for avocadoes that are heavy for their size, and avoid any with soft or dark spots. An avocado is ripe when it yields slightly when pressed at the stem end, and to speed ripening you can put the fruit in a brown paper bag in a warm spot. Once ripe, an avocado can be refrigerated for up to five days. Like a banana, avocado should be added to juices in a blender and not put through the juicer. Yield: 2 ounces of juice per pound of avocado.

Juicy Jive

If you cut open an avocado and it's still unripe, coat the exposed surfaces with mayonnaise, push the avocado back together, and allow it to continue ripening.

Beets. Beets are a "two-fer" of the vegetable bin. You can juice the prized roots and also the leaves as long as they are perky and not wilted. The roots are a good source of calcium, potassium, and iron, while the greens are rich in calcium, iron, and vitamins A and C. Choose beets that are small to medium in size, and a key to selection is that the greens should be fresh. Beets should always be scrubbed well. After all, they did come out of the dirt! When you get beets home, store beets and greens separately. Use the greens within two days, but refrigerate the beets themselves in a plastic bag for up to two weeks. Yield: 6 to 7 ounces per pound of either beets or beet greens.

Wrong Spin!

Never, ever consume beet juice alone, because it can cause a severe inflammation of the throat and esophagus. No juice should ever be more than 50 percent beet juice.

Broccoli. Even broccoli's detractors have to admit that it boasts a strong nutritional profile. A one-cup serving provides the same amount of protein as an equal portion of rice or corn, but with one third of the calories. It's an excellent source of calcium, as well as being very high in antioxidants and vitamins B6, C, and E. Firm stalks, tightly closed bright green heads, and a fresh aroma are the way to select this member of the cruciferous family. Avoid broccoli that has a strong cabbage smell, dried or woody stems, and yellowed florets, and use it within four days to preserve its nutrients. Broccoli has a strong flavor if consumed by itself as a juice. Always wash broccoli well. Grit and even insects or worms can be hiding in the florets. Yield: 6 ounces of juice per pound of broccoli.

Cabbage. There are different types of cabbage, and all are high in vitamin C. Savoy cabbage has wrinkled leaves, while common white cabbage has shiny light green leaves. For both species, select heads that are firm and heavy for their size. Don't select a head that has discolored leaves or feels light, because both are signs it's been picked for some time. Rinse cabbage well, trim the stem end, and store it in the refrigerator for up to two weeks. Always store it in a plastic bag, because some of its natural aroma can transfer to more delicate foods. Yield: 6 ounces of juice per pound of cabbage.

Pulp Tidbits

While native to Afghanistan, carrots were known in Europe long before the Christian Era. Both Greeks and Romans wrote about them but actually preferred turnips for eating.

Carrots. The color is a tip-off that carrots are high in beta-carotene, but they also are excellent sources of vitamins A, B, and C. On the mineral side, they're an excellent source of calcium, phosphorous, potassium, and sodium. It's good to buy carrots that have the lacy foliage attached as a sign of how fresh they are, but discard the foliage as soon as you get them home. Carrot foliage actually robs the carrots of moisture and vitamins if left attached. Pick carrots that are thin, firm, and smooth, and deeply colored. Avoid any with cracks or if they've begun to become soft or wither. Refrigerate carrots for up to a week, but discard them if they begin to show cracks. Yield: 6 to 8 ounces of juice per pound of carrots.

Cauliflower. Like broccoli, cabbage, and other cruciferous veggies, cauliflower by itself can be rather strong, so always mix it with other vegetables and perhaps some fruits. High in vitamin C, cauliflower should be snowy white with no discoloration on the florets when you buy it. Try to use it within four days, although you can refrigerate it for up to a week. Another thing to look for is that leaves are bright green and fresh-looking. Yield: 6 ounces of juice per pound of cauliflower.

Celery. Celery juice is mild in flavor, and its natural sodium content adds to any mixture, so it's one of the most versatile to juice. Pascal is the type of celery we find in American supermarkets, although other varieties are grown around the world. High in vitamin C and potassium, choose celery stalks that are bright green and firm with fresh-looking leaves. Store celery refrigerated for up to a week. Cut off the stem end, separate the ribs, and wash them well. There's always a large amount of dirt embedded at the stem end. For juicing, all you have to do is rinse it well and cut it into 2-inch lengths. Juice the ribs and the leaves, or leave the leaves on the short sprigs to use as a garnish. Yield: 8 to 10 ounces of juice per pound of celery.

> **Juicy Jive**
>
> There's a big difference between the natural sodium found in foods like celery and sodium chloride, or table salt. Natural sodium is alkaline so it balances the pH of the blood and makes the body's use of calcium more effective. Natural sodium makes our blood salty, but it doesn't raise our blood pressure.

Cucumbers. Like celery, the mild taste of cucumbers makes them a foil for more dominant flavors in a juice, and they also pair nicely with herbs. Select cucumbers that are firm, dark green, and have a skin that is slightly bumpy but not wrinkled. Organic cucumbers are never waxed, but should you buy a conventional one, always peel it. Peeling cucumbers is a shame because the skin contains almost all the valuable vitamin A content as well as the mineral silica, which is good for connective tissue and your complexion. Use cucumbers within four days after picking. Yield: 8 ounces of juice per pound of unpeeled cucumbers.

Fennel. Americans are just beginning to appreciate the wonders of fennel, a vegetable similar to celery with a nutritional profile that is high in sodium, calcium, and magnesium. Its slight mild licorice flavor makes a wonderful juice that blends with stronger vegetables and fruits. Fennel is basically a winter vegetable, and it's at its peak from November to April. Pick fennel bulbs that are about the size of tennis balls and show no bruising or discoloration on the skin, store them refrigerated, and use them within five days. For juicing, use both the bulb and stalks, and save the feathery greens for a garnish. Trim off the stem end, rinse the bulb, and cut it into pieces to fit your juicer. Yield: 6 to 8 ounces of juice per pound of fennel.

> **Juicy Jive**
>
> The species of fennel we use for juicing as well as cooking is the Italian strain sometimes referred to as Florence fennel; it's also just called fresh anise in some supermarkets.

Garlic. This bulbous member of the lily family is a wonder food that has been proven to reduce cholesterol as well as the risk of heart disease. Available year-round, choose heads that are firm and not dry or shriveled, and store them in a cool, dry place. Don't refrigerate garlic, because it will cause it to sprout. If you see green shoots emerging from the tips of the cloves, don't buy them; they indicate that it's old and sprouting. It's best to store garlic in a cool, dry place and not refrigerate it. Yield: Only used for flavoring, and usually 1 or 2 cloves is sufficient.

Ginger. While we refer to ginger as a root, it's actually a *rhizome* native to Asia that has a sweet and somewhat peppery flavor. When choosing ginger, look for nodules that are large, firm, and have a shiny skin. Avoid ones that are dull and shriveled. Store it refrigerated for up to a week. It's not necessary to peel ginger for juicing, so the size of the bulb doesn't matter, but for general cooking, select large pieces or you'll peel away the majority. Yield: Only used for flavoring, and most juice recipes call for 2 to 4 tablespoons of sliced ginger.

> **Liquid Lingo**
>
> A **rhizome** is different from a root. It's actually an underground part of the stem that usually grows horizontally. Ginger is an edible rhizome, but many exist in nature.

Kale. Kale is the renegade cousin of the cabbage clan. Rather than growing as a compact head or with tight florets, it grows like a bouquet of flowers. It's very high in iron as well as vitamins A, B, and C. Choose heads with crisp, dark green leaves, and pass by heads that have even a tinge of yellow in the leaves or are limp. Refrigerate it loosely in a plastic bag for up to five days. Kale is easy to juice. Just rinse it well, and break it into lengths that fit into your juicer. Yield: 6 ounces of juice per pound of fennel.

Parsnips. These iron-colored vegetables are first cousins of the carrots, and both have an essentially sweet flavor, although the flavor of parsnips is somewhat stronger. Choose large parsnips that are very firm, and look for feathery tops, which you should discard as soon as they arrive home. Like carrots, store parsnips for up to a week. Parsnips are a good source of vitamin C and also contain large amounts of potassium, phosphorous, and silicon. Yield: 4 ounces of juice per pound of parsnips.

> **Juicy Jive**
>
> Parsnips are sometimes harder to find than ubiquitous carrots, so feel free to substitute carrots for them anytime you're juicing. Be aware, however, that the color of the juice might not be as pleasing.

Peppers, bell. Bell peppers, a good source of vitamin C, are best if they're allowed to ripen on the vine. That's why red peppers, which are also high in vitamin A, are so much sweeter than green peppers, which are just immature. When choosing peppers, look for ones that are firm and shiny, and avoid ones that are shriveled. Store refrigerated but not in plastic bags for up to a week. For juicing, remove the cap and pull out the large clump of seeds, although you don't have to be meticulous about seed removal. Then rinse the pepper, at which time more seeds will fall off, and cut it into pieces to fit your juicer. Yield: 5 to 6 ounces of juice per pound of peppers.

Potatoes. Potatoes add a light flavor to juices, and they're high in vitamin C and several of the B vitamins, as well as potassium. If pulped instead of juiced, they are also a good source of soluble fiber. Choose potatoes that are firm and free from blemishes, discolorations, or sprouting eyes. Yield: 3 ounces of juice per pound of potatoes.

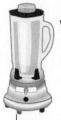

Wrong Spin!

If you get a potato home and discover that it has a green cast to the flesh, throw it out. The green indicates the presence of solanine, a toxin caused if potatoes are exposed to light when growing.

Scallions. You'll notice that scallions, also called green onions, are the member of this offshoot of the lily family I use most often for juices. And the reason is simple. They are the mildest, and their delicate flavor blends well with myriad vegetables. They are also about the same size, so you don't have to "guesstimate" what is small or large. Scallions should be firm with unblemished bulbs and perky green tops, so avoid ones that are limp. Most scallions will start to go limp after three or four days of refrigeration. Yield: 2 ounces of juice per pound of scallions.

Spinach. Popeye was right: spinach is a wonder food. It's a great source of iron, phosphorous, and fiber as well as vitamins A, B, C, E, and K. It's best to buy loose spinach rather than in bags so you can really see the condition of the leaves, which should be crisp, firm, and dark green. Also choose a bunch with short stems. Store it refrigerated for up to four days. Give spinach a very careful washing, and follow with a second bath if the leaves are very dirty. Spinach doesn't produce all that much juice when compared to its bulk, so I don't use it very often, but if you prefer to drink it rather than eat it as a salad, juice away! Yield: 4 ounces of juice per pound of spinach.

Wrong Spin!

Don't believe those bags that say that vegetables or lettuce has been pre-washed. They might have given you a leg up on the process, but the job's not done. I've done numerous tests and always find lingering dirt. I don't like to wash tender greens in a salad spinner because it can bruise or break them. For those vegetables, swish them around in a large bowl of cold water, rubbing stem ends with your fingers. Then remove them from the bowl and pat them dry with paper towels. And look at the amount of grit in the bottom of the bowl from your pre-washed produce!

Tomatoes. Botanists classify tomatoes as a fruit, but I'm listing them in the vegetable section because we eat them as a vegetable. Today's science touts tomatoes for their lycopene content, which is proven to have anti-cancer qualities. In addition, they contain a good amount of vitamin C and potassium. There's nothing like a vine-ripened tomato fresh from the garden. Second to that, choose ones at the market that don't have ridges at the stem end, which is a sign the tomato might be mealy, and always choose the brightest red possible. If ripe, refrigerate them for up to four days. While tomatoes—like most fruits—do ripen once they're picked, the flavor is never as sweet as if they're allowed to stay on their fragrant vines in the field. If you live anywhere near a farmer's market, I suggest you buy them there. Yield: 8 to 10 ounces of juice per pound of tomatoes.

Sweet Potatoes/Yams. These two vegetables, both high in carotenes, vitamin C, calcium, and potassium, are decidedly different species, but I'm lumping them together because of their similarity in taste and because you can substitute one for another at any time. Look for tubers that are firm, shiny, and fresh-looking, and avoid ones that are shriveled. Store them in a cool, dry place. Scrub well before juicing, but there's no need to peel them. Yield: 4 ounces of juice per pound of sweet potatoes or yams.

Zucchini. This mild-tasting member of the summer squash family is a good source of vitamins A and C, potassium, and niacin. Choose small zucchini that are unblemished and firm, and refrigerate them for up to five days in a plastic bag. Substitute yellow crookneck squash for zucchini in any juice recipe, and even the color will not change because zucchini juice is such a pale green. Yield: 8 ounces of juice per pound of zucchini.

Pulp Tidbits

Sweet potatoes bolster Thor Heyerdahl's theory that natives of South America succeeded in crossing the Pacific Ocean. The Maoris of New Zealand have a tradition that the sweet potato, native to the Americas, reached them from the country of their ancestors.

The Least You Need to Know

◆ Vegetables do not ripen like fruits and should be eaten as soon as possible after they've been picked.

◆ Always mix beet juice with other ingredients and never consume it by itself.

◆ Broccoli contains the same amount of protein as corn or rice but with one third of the calories.

◆ Garlic reduces "bad" cholesterol.

◆ Tomatoes are actually a fruit, although we eat them like a vegetable.

Chapter 4

Added Attractions

In This Chapter

- ◆ Soy foods
- ◆ Dietary supplements
- ◆ Herbs for aroma and flavor
- ◆ Juices in other forms

Fruits and vegetables are the stars of the juice world, but as in every recipe, you also need supporting players. In this chapter, you'll learn what your options are for those "extra" ingredients.

If you want to add a little extra nutritional kick to your juice, you'll learn which nutritional supplements the vivid flavors of your fresh juices can best mask.

To dress up juices for parties or just for the fun of it, you can easily make a number of garnishes to sit on the rim of the glass. Those tips and ideas are in this chapter, too.

The Joy of Soy

No wonder they call soy a wonder food! Lately, researchers are discovering more and more nutritional benefits from soy products. For example, soybeans are the only known plant source of *complete protein.* In addition, the Food and Drug Administration (FDA) has approved a health claim stating that diets containing 25 grams of soy protein a day may reduce the risk of heart disease.

> **Liquid Lingo**
>
> **Complete protein** is the term used for a food that contains all the essential amino acids in the appropriate proportions that are part of the growth and maintenance of cells. Meats and some dairy products have complete protein, while grains and beans contain incomplete proteins. Blending incomplete proteins, such as rice and beans, produces a complete protein. But in the plant world, soy alone has it all.

In addition, soy is low-fat, and products made from soy create great juices. Here are a few:

Soy milk. This nondairy "milk" is made by grinding soybeans to a flourlike consistency, cooking the flour with water, and pressing out the liquid. Soy milk is rich in protein and iron, and most manufacturers fortify their soy milk with calcium as well. Whole and low-fat versions are also available. Use soy milk interchangeably with dairy milk in any recipe.

> **Wrong Spin!**
>
> Although you can blend any form of tofu into your juices, do not substitute tempeh for tofu. Tempeh is made from fermented soybeans, and its crumbly texture and savory flavor are not really compatible with many vegetables or fruits.

Silken tofu. Tofu is a curd made from pressed and drained soybeans and comes in a number of densities, such as firm and silken, depending on how hard it was pressed during manufacture. Tofu is high in B vitamins, potassium, and iron, and some tofu is also high in calcium, if that mineral was used as the curdling agent. The best tofu for juices is silken tofu because it adds a soft texture to the drink. If you're using a firmer tofu, you might want to add additional liquid to the blender.

Powerful Powders

You can easily turn a juice into an energy- and nutrient-packed meal by just adding a few tablespoons of a nutritional supplement for additional protein, vitamins, and minerals. You should be able to find most of these supplements in many grocery and most health food stores. They are not specified in the recipes in this book, but you can add any of them to any juice concoction.

Bee pollen. Bee pollen is made from the seeds of flower blossoms that stick to the bees' legs as they're going about their tasks. When they return to their hive, they clean their legs, mixing these seeds with nectar and their own enzymes to form the pollen. It's rich with protein; vitamins A, B, C, and E; as well as calcium and magnesium. Bee pollen doesn't change the taste of juices at all, so add up to 2 tablespoons to any juice recipe.

Flaxseed. Flaxseed is the best vegetable source for essential omega-3 fatty acids, the same beneficial fat found in salmon and other fish. Flaxseed also contains lecithin, which aids in digestion. The seeds have to be ground up to release their benefits, so put up to 2 tablespoons into any juice recipe and blend away. Flaxseed does have a nutty flavor, but it will probably be masked by other ingredients in the juice.

Soy protein powder. There are protein powders on the market made from cow's milk or eggs, but the most popular is a flavorless powder with all the health benefits of soybeans. The texture of some brands tends to be a bit grainy, but you can add 2 or 3 tablespoons per juice recipe, and the texture from the other ingredients will mask that of the powder.

Wheat germ. Wheat germ is the embryo of a wheat berry, and adding just 1 tablespoon to a juice recipe adds 2 grams of protein and 1 gram of fiber.

> ### Juicy Jive
>
> It's best to add all nutritional supplements to juices at the beginning of the blending process. Some, such as flaxseed and wheat germ, benefit from being puréed well while other ingredients are added to the blender.

Wheat germ has a slightly nutty flavor. It's an exceptional source of vitamin E and also contains thiamin and copper. Add up to 2 tablespoons per recipe—or more if you like the nutty flavor.

Herbal Additions

Fresh herbs add anticipatory aroma as well as fresh flavor to all foods, including juices. Botanically an herb is the leaf of specific plants, most of which grow in temperate climates.

It's easy to grow fresh herbs in your garden, and the aroma and flavor is never as good as the moment they're picked. Even if you live in an apartment, you can grow small pots of herbs on a sunny window sill.

The recipes in Chapter 7 are devoted to juices that star herbs along with vegetables and even the occasional fruit. But you can add herbs to any vegetable juice. Here is a list of frequently used herbs:

Basil. Now more popular than ever garnishing many Italian dishes and as the main ingredient in pesto, basil has a pungent flavor and aroma that's almost a cross between anise and cloves. Choose bunches with bright leaves that aren't wilted.

Chives. Chives are related to onions and leeks and have a very mild onion flavor. They're long and green and can be snipped to any length with a pair of scissors.

Cilantro. Cilantro, sometimes called fresh coriander or Chinese parsley, was almost unknown in this country until the 1980s when both regional American and ethnic cooking began to grow. It has a pungent aroma and flavor, and many consider it an acquired taste. It's used extensively in Mexican, Southwestern, and Asian cooking.

Dill. This fresh-tasting herb has feathery bright green leaves that look similar to those of fennel and is used extensively in Scandinavian cooking for such dishes as Gravlax and Swedish Meatballs. It's also used in Greek dishes.

Mint. Mint will take over a garden, so relegate it to a pot if you're growing herbs. Two species of mint are widely available. Peppermint is the more pungent of the two and has bright green leaves. Spearmint, with gray-green leaves, is more delicate in aroma and color.

Oregano. This herb, popular in Mediterranean cooking, is a member of the mint family but is also related to both thyme and marjoram. It adds a pungent aroma and almost spicy flavor to juices.

Parsley. Long before any other herbs began appearing in produce sections, cooks could always find a bunch of fresh-tasting parsley. In addition to using it in cooking, parsley's probably the most ubiquitous garnish in the country if not on the planet.

Rosemary. Rosemary is another mint family cousin, and its long, bright green needles convey the aroma of pine with a slight flavor of lemon. It's native to the Mediterranean region and is used in many European cuisines.

> **Juicy Jive**
>
> While there are more than 30 types of parsley, the most common ones are curly and Italian flat-leaf. Most cooks prefer the latter because it is more strongly flavored, but either can be used. Until a few years ago flat-leaf parsley was harder to find, but all supermarkets now carry both.

Tarragon. Tarragon is one of the stalwarts of classic French cooking. It has a pungent anise aroma and flavor that blends very well with grassy vegetables like celery and asparagus.

Great Garnishes

You might think it's crazy to garnish a juice. After all, you've already got a glass of a food with a delicious taste and (most of the time) a vivid color.

But occasionally you might have a few extra minutes and want to make the juice more special. Or maybe it's a special occasion and you want to elicit a "Wow!" when you serve the frosty glasses. Whatever your reason, garnish away! I've annotated each recipe with a suggested garnish, but you can ignore those suggestions and add any of these:

Fruit kebabs. Kebabs are the no-brainer of garnishes. Reserve some of the fruit used in the juice and thread bite-size pieces onto a toothpick or a little plastic sword that doubles as a toothpick. For a fancier look, use a few different types of fruit.

Strawberry "fans." Reserve the large strawberries from your box for the garnish before you purée the rest. Rinse the berries, but do not remove the green cap. Using a sharp paring knife, make five or six cuts through the berry, starting at the cap. Transfer the strawberry to a plate, and gently push apart the slices to form a fan.

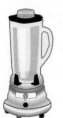

> **Wrong Spin!**
>
> Herbs like rosemary, sage, and thyme are not appropriate for garnishes because the stems are too woody. Pull the leaves off the stems of all these herbs before using.

Herb sprigs. Any delicate herb, such as parsley, cilantro, mint, or dill, makes a pretty and edible garnish. Rinse the sprig, and tuck it on the side of the glass.

Culinary Creations

It's always nice to know that a piece of kitchen equipment can do double duty, and that's the case with juicers and blenders. While intended for drinks to quaff immediately, they can be useful in other ways.

You'll find criteria for selecting and using both juicers and blenders in Chapter 1 of this book. This section is intended to give you reasons to keep them on the counter.

Smooth Sailing

The basic difference between a juice and a smoothie is the texture. Smoothies are always thick because some of the ingredients are frozen.

It's easy to turn a juice into a smoothie by taking some of the juice and freezing it in ice cube trays. The proportion should be about half and half frozen and chilled. Then place the juice in a blender and turn it on high. In about 30 seconds you'll have a thick, frosty juice drink. But don't use ice cubes made from water or it will dilute the juice too much.

Freezing does lessen some of the nutrients culled from the juice ingredients, but most of them are preserved.

Great Granitas

To make a smoothie, freeze only half of the juice, but if you take the process further, the juice can become a *granita*. Serve these ices in myriad ways. Place a dollop on top of a chilled summer soup, serve it as a palate cleanser between courses, or place it on top of fresh fruit as a dessert.

The easy way to make granita is to freeze all the juice in ice cube trays until it is about 75 percent frozen. Then place the cubes in a food processor fitted with a steel blade, and pulse it on and off until it becomes mushy.

Return the mixture to the freezer in a mixing bowl. Once it has become frozen again, it's ready to use. Remove the granita to soften 20 minutes before serving it.

> **Liquid Lingo**
>
> **Granita** is hard like granite, but it's the Italian word for ice. The term is used to describe any hard, granular frozen ice that can be either sweet or savory.

Gourmet Gelatin

Vegetable and fruit aspics are nothing more than juices thickened by gelatin. While they were very popular back in the 1960s, they fell from favor with devoted foodies. But like many foods, such as fondue, they're beginning to make a comeback in popularity.

Juicers make a mean aspic. The general rule of thumb is to use one ¼-ounce package of granulated gelatin for every 2 cups of liquid. The first step is to soak the granules in cold liquid for 3 to 5 minutes so they will soften and swell up. This makes them dissolve smoothly when heated.

> **Pulp Tidbits**
>
> Commercial gelatin didn't hit the scene until the late nineteenth century. Until then cooks had to make their own by laboriously boiling calves' feet. The only other products that produced the desired effect were isinglass, which is a natural gelatin from fish air bladders, or carrageen, a dried seaweed. Most commercial gelatin today is a by-product of pig skin.

Heat the juice until the gelatin dissolves, and then chill it until firm in a mold or bowl.

Other Ideas

You'll find that your juicer can become a useful piece of equipment for everyday cooking as well as juicing. All those trimmings and scraps you are now throwing into the garbage after prepping vegetables for dishes might be candidates to be pushed through the juicer to intensify the flavor of the dish you're cooking.

For example, if you're making a dish with asparagus—like an asparagus risotto or cream of asparagus soup—chances are you'll throw away the woody parts of the stems. But you can put them through the juicer and then use the resulting juice for part of the liquid specified in your recipe. The same holds true for any recipe made with broccoli.

Are you making a pot of vegetable soup? Push the well-washed carrot scrapings and celery trimmings through the juicer. While the nutrients will be lost through cooking, you'll boost the flavor.

The Least You Need to Know

- ◆ Soybeans provide complete protein in the diet.
- ◆ Add nutritional supplements to any juice to turn it into a complete meal.
- ◆ Store fresh herbs in the refrigerator and freeze some of them.
- ◆ Transform juices into smoothies or granitas by freezing some or all of the juice.

2

Garden Patch Purées

Noshing various elements from a platter of crudité is the same principle as making the juices from the recipes in this part. The difference is that you push the various elements through the juicer or pulp them in the blender.

Juices are an easy and delicious way to fulfill that hard-to-meet guideline of eating seven servings of vegetables a day. In this part you'll find recipes with great combinations of different vegetables—with a fruit thrown in, too.

5

The Root of the Matter

In This Chapter

- ◆ Juices made with bright orange carrots
- ◆ Delicate juices sweetened by pale parsnips
- ◆ Ruby red juices based on beets

Root vegetables, such as carrots, parsnips, and beets, are nature's candy store because they are sweet right out of the ground and need little embellishment. And for these reasons, they're the stars of the recipes in this chapter.

But their dynamite flavor is too much of a good thing if taken alone. Many people have adverse reactions to juices made from just root vegetables. This caution leads to complex flavors as these stars are joined by delicious supporting players.

Tapping Out

These three vegetables all fall under the umbrella of taproots for biennial plants. The biennial part means that a plant only lives for two years, and then you must plant a new patch.

The reason why carrots, parsnips, and beets are all so inherently sweet is that sugar must be stored up in the root to allow the plant to flower and grow for a second year. Indeed, carrots actually put forth lovely delicate white blossoms that chefs use to garnish plates when available.

But there is some variation amongst the taproot clan. The beet greens that are visible above the ground are as tasty in their own way as the beet itself. But the leaves giving life to carrots and parsnips are for decoration only, and you should totally discard them before juicing their roots.

Carrot and Asparagus

4 carrots

½ lb. asparagus

4 celery ribs

2 apples

2 cups firmly packed spinach leaves

2 carrot sticks for garnish (optional)

Serves 2
Prep time: less than 10 minutes
Each serving: 162 calories 9 calories from fat 1 g fat 0 g saturated fat 5 g protein 38 g carbohydrates

1. Scrub carrots, discard green tops, and cut into 2-inch lengths. Rinse asparagus and cut into 2-inch lengths. Rinse celery and cut into 2-inch lengths. Rinse apples and cut into sixths. Rinse spinach leaves.

2. Push carrots, asparagus, celery, apples, and spinach through the juicer, and process until juiced. Stir well and pour juice into two glasses.

3. Serve immediately, garnished with carrot sticks if desired.

Variation: To pulp this recipe in a blender or food processor fitted with a steel blade, core apple and cut all ingredients into pieces no larger than 1 inch.

Juicy Jive

The reason we add celery to so many juices is that it's a great natural source of sodium. The sodium perks the flavor of the other ingredients the way adding table salt to food enhances flavors, but in a natural way.

Fruity Carrot

4 carrots

2 apples

2 oranges

1 cup red seedless grapes

½ cup raspberries

¼ lime

2 lime wedges for garnish (optional)

Serves 2
Prep time: less than 10 minutes
Each serving: 258 calories 9 calories from fat 1 g fat 0 g saturated fat 4 g protein 66 g carbohydrates

1. Scrub carrots, discard green tops, and cut into 2-inch lengths. Rinse apples and cut into sixths. Peel oranges and cut into quarters. Rinse grapes and raspberries, and peel lime.

2. Push carrots, apples, oranges, grapes, raspberries, and lime through the juicer, and process until juiced. Stir well and pour juice into two glasses.

3. Serve immediately, garnished with lime wedges if desired.

Variation: To pulp this recipe in a blender or food processor fitted with a steel blade, core apples and cut all ingredients into pieces no larger than 1 inch.

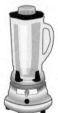

Wrong Spin!

Literally hundreds of species of apples are grown, and what's important for juicing is not the name of the apple but its flavor. Certain apples, such as Granny Smiths, need to be sweetened with sugar for baking. The best apples for juicing are McIntosh, Golden Delicious, or Rome.

Tropical Carrot

4 carrots

2 celery ribs

2 apples

1 mango

¼ lime

1½ cups peeled and cubed pineapple

2 lime wedges for garnish (optional)

Serves 2
Prep time: less than 10 minutes
Each serving: 254 calories 9 calories from fat 1 g fat 0 g saturated fat 3 g protein 66 g carbohydrates

1. Scrub carrots, discard green tops, and cut into 2-inch lengths. Rinse celery and cut into 2-inch lengths. Rinse apples and cut into sixths. Peel mango and cut fruit away from seed. Peel lime.

2. Push carrots, apples, celery, mango, lime, and pineapple through the juicer, and process until juiced. Stir well and pour juice into two glasses.

3. Serve immediately, garnished with lime wedges if desired.

Variation: To pulp this recipe in a blender or food processor fitted with a steel blade, *core* apples, remove seeds from lime, and cut all ingredients into pieces no larger than 1 inch.

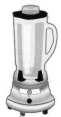

Wrong Spin!

Few fruits are as luscious as a ripe mango. But few fruits are as awful as a rock-hard one. If all you can find is a green, hard mango, then substitute papaya in the recipe. Mangoes do ripen faster if placed in a brown paper bag with some apples.

Carrot Kale

6 carrots

4 celery ribs

1 apple

3 cups firmly packed kale leaves

½ tsp. celery seed

2 celery sprigs for garnish (optional)

Serves 2
Prep time: less than 10 minutes
Each serving: 177 calories 18 calories from fat 2 g fat 0 g saturated fat 6 g protein 40 g carbohydrates

1. Scrub carrots, discard green tops, and cut into 2-inch lengths. Rinse celery and cut into 2-inch lengths. Rinse apples and cut into sixths. Rinse kale leaves, and cut into 2-inch lengths.

2. Push carrots, celery, apple, and kale leaves through the juicer, and process until juiced. Pour juice into two glasses. Stir ¼ teaspoon celery seed into each glass.

3. Serve immediately, garnished with celery sprigs if desired.

Variation: To pulp this recipe in a blender or food processor fitted with a steel blade, core apple and cut all ingredients into pieces no larger than 1 inch.

Liquid Lingo ⸻

Core is both a noun and a verb. As a noun it's the woody center of fruit such as apples and pears that contains hard, indigestible seeds. The verb means to remove and discard these elements.

Carrot Jicama

4 carrots

2 celery ribs

3 cups firmly packed spinach leaves

$^1/_2$ jicama

$^1/_2$ cup silken tofu

Pinch of ground nutmeg

2 slices jicama for garnish (optional)

Serves 2
Prep time: less than 10 minutes
Each serving: 163 calories 9 calories from fat 1 g fat 0 g saturated fat 5 g protein 35 g carbohydrates

1. Scrub carrots, discard green tops, and cut into 2-inch lengths. Rinse celery and cut into 2-inch lengths. Rinse spinach leaves. Rinse jicama and cut into 2-inch cubes.

2. Push carrots, celery, spinach, and jicama through the juicer, and process until juiced. Pour juice into a blender and add tofu and nutmeg. Blend for 30 seconds. Pour juice into two glasses.

3. Serve immediately, garnished with jicama slices if desired.

Variation: To pulp this recipe in a blender or food processor fitted with a steel blade, peel jicama and cut all ingredients into pieces no larger than 1 inch. If using a blender or food processor, add tofu and nutmeg along with other ingredients.

Pulp Tidbits

Nutmeg was one of the reasons Columbus discovered America. Nutmeg is the seed of a tropical evergreen native to the Spice Islands that was most popular with European aristocracy beginning in the fifteenth century. When the fruit of the tree is split, it reveals the inch-long nutmeg seed surrounded by a lacy membrane that is ground into mace, a spice similar in flavor.

Spiced Carrot, Pineapple, and Banana

6 carrots

¼ lime

3 ripe bananas

½ ripe pineapple

½ tsp. Chinese five-spice powder

2 pineapple spears for garnish (optional)

Serves 2
Prep time: less than 10 minutes
Each serving: 304 calories 9 calories from fat 1 g fat 0 g saturated fat 4 g protein 76 g carbohydrates

1. Scrub carrots, discard green tops, and cut into 2-inch lengths. Peel lime. Peel and slice bananas. Cut the pineapple off its rind and cut it into 2-inch cubes.

2. Push carrots, pineapple, and lime through the juicer, and process until juiced. Pour juice into a blender, and add bananas and *Chinese five-spice powder*. Blend for 30 seconds. Stir well and pour juice into two glasses.

3. Serve immediately, garnished with pineapple spears if desired.

Variation: To pulp this recipe in a blender or food processor fitted with a steel blade, remove seeds from lime and cut all ingredients into pieces no larger than 1 inch. If using a blender or food processor, add bananas and five-spice powder along with other ingredients.

Liquid Lingo ———

Chinese five-spice powder is perhaps the oldest blend of spices around. Having been used in traditional Chinese cooking for centuries, it's made up of equal parts cinnamon, cloves, fennel seed, star anise, and Szechwan peppercorns. It's available in most supermarkets, found either with spices or with Asian food.

Parsnip and Lettuce

6 parsnips

2 celery ribs

2 scallions

3 cups firmly packed green leaf lettuce

¼ cup firmly packed parsley sprigs

Freshly ground black pepper to taste

2 celery sprigs for garnish (optional)

Serves 2
Prep time: less than 10 minutes
Each serving: 371 calories 18 calories from fat 2 g fat 0 g saturated fat 8 g protein 88 g carbohydrates

1. Scrub parsnips, discard green tops, and cut into 2-inch lengths. Rinse celery and cut into 2-inch lengths. Trim scallions and cut into 2-inch lengths. Rinse lettuce leaves, cut into 2-inch lengths, and rinse parsley sprigs.

2. Push parsnips, celery, scallions, lettuce, and parsley through the juicer, and process until juiced. Stir well and pour juice into two glasses. Season each glass to taste with pepper.

3. Serve immediately, garnished with celery sprigs if desired.

Variation: To pulp this recipe in a blender or food processor fitted with a steel blade, core apple and cut all ingredients into pieces no larger than 1 inch.

Juicy Jive

Ingredients that are light and bulky, like fresh herbs and lettuce leaves, should always be firmly packed into a measuring cup to gauge an accurate amount. That's why fresh herbs in most recipes are chopped before measuring, but that's a waste of time when the whole sprigs are about to go into a juicer or blender.

Spiced Parsnip and Tomato

4 parsnips

4 celery ribs

8 ripe plum tomatoes

¼ tsp. ground coriander

¼ tsp. ground cumin

Freshly ground black pepper to taste

2 tomato wedges for garnish (optional)

Serves 2

Prep time:
less than 10 minutes

Each serving:
345 calories
27 calories from fat
3 g fat
0 g saturated fat
9 g protein
80 g carbohydrates

1. Scrub parsnips, discard green tops, and cut into 2-inch lengths. Rinse celery and cut into 2-inch lengths. Rinse tomatoes and cut into quarters.

2. Push parsnips, celery, and tomatoes through the juicer, and process until juiced. Pour juice into two glasses. Stir ⅛ teaspoon coriander and ⅛ teaspoon cumin into each glass, and season to taste with pepper.

3. Serve immediately, garnished with tomato wedges if desired.

Variation: To pulp this recipe in a blender or food processor fitted with a steel blade, cut all ingredients into pieces no larger than 1 inch and add coriander and cumin along with other ingredients.

Pulp Tidbits

Ground coriander is the seed from the same plant that produces cilantro as fresh leaves, although the flavor is totally different. Coriander is one of the world's earliest recorded ingredients. The seeds themselves were discovered in an Egyptian tomb that dates from 960 B.C.E.

Parsnip and Fennel

6 parsnips

2 celery ribs

2 scallions

1 fennel bulb

Freshly ground black pepper to taste

2 celery sprigs for garnish (optional)

Serves 2
Prep time: less than 10 minutes
Each serving: 391 calories 18 calories from fat 2 g fat 0 g saturated fat 8 g protein 93 g carbohydrates

1. Scrub parsnips, discard green tops, and cut into 2-inch lengths. Rinse celery and cut into 2-inch lengths. Rinse scallions and cut into 2-inch lengths. Rinse fennel bulb, trim stem end, and cut into 2-inch cubes.

2. Push parsnips, celery, scallions, and *fennel* through the juicer, and process until juiced. Stir well and pour juice into two glasses. Season each glass to taste with pepper.

3. Serve immediately, garnished with celery sprigs if desired.

Variation: To pulp this recipe in a blender or food processor fitted with a steel blade, trim scallions and cut all ingredients into pieces no larger than 1 inch.

Liquid Lingo

Fennel is a plant native to the Mediterranean that looks like celery, but has a mild anise flavor (like black licorice). While it's called finocchio in Italian markets, it's also called fresh anise in many supermarkets. You can use the stalks raw in place of celery in salads, and the bulb can be eaten raw, stir-fried, or braised in stock.

Gingered Sesame Beet and Yam

2 beets

2 carrots

1 yam

1 apple

2 scallions

3 TB. sliced fresh ginger

2 TB. tahini paste

2 apple wedges for garnish (optional)

Serves 2

Prep time:
less than 10 minutes

Each serving:
285 calories
81 calories from fat
9 g fat
1 g saturated fat
6 g protein
49 g carbohydrates

1. Scrub beets well, discard tops if wilted but rinse and use if not, and cut into 2-inch cubes. Scrub carrots, discard green tops, and cut into 2-inch lengths. Scrub yam and cut into 2-inch cubes. Rinse apple and cut into sixths. Rinse scallions and cut into 2-inch lengths.

2. Push beets, carrots, yam, apple, scallions, and ginger through the juicer, and process until juiced. Pour juice into a blender, and add tahini paste. Blend for 30 seconds. Pour juice into two glasses.

3. Serve immediately, garnished with apple wedges if desired.

Variation: To pulp this recipe in a blender or food processor fitted with a steel blade, core apple, trim scallions, and cut all ingredients into pieces no larger than 1 inch. If using a blender or food processor, add tahini paste along with other ingredients.

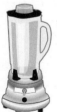

Wrong Spin!

Tahini paste is made from ground sesame seeds, and the oil has a tendency to separate in the container. Be sure to stir it well before measuring. You may have to transfer it to a mixing bowl to stir if the container is very full.

Minted Beet and Wheatgrass

2 oz. wheatgrass

2 large or 4 small beets

2 oranges

2 TB. fresh mint leaves

2 mint sprigs for garnish (optional)

Serves 2
Prep time:
less than 10 minutes
Each serving:
144 calories
4 calories from fat
0.5 g fat
0 g saturated fat
5 g protein
33 g carbohydrates

1. Extract juice from wheatgrass in a wheatgrass juicer, and set aside. Alternately, pureé wheatgrass with ¹/₂ cup water in a blender.

2. Scrub beets well, discard tops if wilted but rinse and use if not, and cut into 2-inch cubes. Peel oranges and cut into quarters.

3. Push beets, oranges, and mint leaves through the juicer, and process until juiced.

4. Pour juice into two glasses, and divide wheatgrass juice evenly between them. Stir well and serve immediately, garnished with mint sprigs if desired.

Variation: To pulp this recipe in a blender or food processor fitted with a steel blade, remove seeds from oranges and cut all ingredients into pieces no larger than 1 inch.

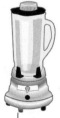

Wrong Spin!

When it comes to wheatgrass, more of something good might not be wonderful. People not used to including this wonder food in their diets may become nauseous if ingesting more than 1 ounce a day due to introducing wheatgrass enzymes into the diet. So start slowly.

6

Drinks from the Cabbage Patch

In This Chapter

- ◆ Refreshing cabbage juices
- ◆ Broccoli juices with bold flavors
- ◆ Colorful juices with cauliflower

The cabbage patch kids suffer from negative public relations. People don't like the way the house smells after they're cooked or their flavors are too strong. I jest, but neither factor is relevant when it comes to juicing!

No aroma lingers from cabbage when juicing because no cooking is involved. Additionally, the flavors are more delicate when eaten raw, and they're always balanced by those of other ingredients. Amongst the recipes in this chapter, you'll find a number of creative cabbage combinations.

The Cruciferous Cousins

Plants are like people. They are related by families, and all plants in the cabbage family fall into the cruciferous clan. This term refers to the small cross shape which is formed when the flowers are growing.

In eras before air importation made it possible for us to eat whatever we wanted regardless of season, cabbages and their cousins were one of the mainstays of winter vegetables. The family includes cabbage, broccoli, cauliflower, kale, and new introductions such as broccoflower, which is a genetically engineered hybrid of broccoli and cauliflower.

The importance of the cabbage clan for our diets is from the high amounts of sulphurophane they contain. Sulphurophane is a compound touted for its anti-cancer properties. This compound was discovered when the diets of East Germany and West Germany were compared during the Cold War. East Germans were poorer, and cabbage consumption was high. The rate of cancer in the country was much lower than that of the more prosperous West Germans.

Cabbage and Jerusalem Artichoke

¼ head green cabbage (about ½ lb.)

2 Jerusalem artichokes

2 celery ribs

3 parsnips

1 cup firmly packed spinach leaves

3 scallions

1 sprig tarragon

2 sprigs tarragon for garnish (optional)

Serves 2
Prep time: less than 10 minutes
Each serving: 262 calories 9 calories from fat 1 g fat 0 g saturated fat 8 g protein 61 g carbohydrates

1. Rinse cabbage, trim stem end, and cut into 2-inch cubes. Scrub Jerusalem artichokes, and cut into 2-inch cubes. Rinse celery and cut into 2-inch lengths. Scrub parsnips, discard green tops, and cut into 2-inch lengths. Rinse spinach. Rinse scallions and cut into 2-inch lengths.

2. Push cabbage, Jerusalem artichokes, celery, parsnips, spinach, scallions, and tarragon through the juicer, and process until juiced. Stir well and pour juice into two glasses.

3. Serve immediately, garnished with tarragon sprigs if desired.

Variation: To pulp this recipe in a blender or food processor fitted with a steel blade, peel Jerusalem artichokes, trim scallions, and cut all ingredients into pieces no larger than 1 inch.

Pulp Tidbits

Jerusalem artichokes are not related to the common globe artichoke, nor do they have anything to do with Jerusalem. They are actually a variety of sunflower, and the name comes from the Italian word for sunflower, *girasole*. You'll see them marketed as Sunchokes in many markets.

Garlicky Cabbage and Turnip

¼ head green cabbage (about ½ lb.)

½ large turnip or 1 small turnip

1 parsnip

3 scallions

¼ cup firmly packed cilantro sprigs

3 garlic cloves

2 cilantro sprigs for garnish (optional)

Serves 2
Prep time: less than 10 minutes
Each serving: 113 calories 5 calories from fat 0.5 g fat 0 g saturated fat 4 g protein 26 g carbohydrates

1. Rinse cabbage, trim stem end, and cut into 2-inch cubes. Scrub turnip and cut into 2-inch cubes. Scrub parsnip, discard green tops, and cut into 2-inch lengths. Rinse scallions and cut into 2-inch lengths. Rinse cilantro sprigs and garlic cloves.

2. Push cabbage, turnip, parsnip, scallions, cilantro, and garlic through the juicer, and process until juiced. Stir well and pour juice into two glasses.

3. Serve immediately, garnished with cilantro sprigs if desired.

Variation: To pulp this recipe in a blender or food processor fitted with a steel blade, peel turnip, trim scallions, peel garlic cloves, and cut all ingredients into pieces no larger than 1 inch.

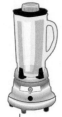

Wrong Spin! _____

Of all the convenience products on the market, perhaps one of the worst is pre-minced garlic. It comes packed in both oil and water, and you should always avoid using it because the flavor isn't good. On the other hand, some supermarkets carry small packages of whole garlic cloves that are pre-peeled. These are great, and you can use them in any recipe.

Cabbage, Spinach, and Celery

¼ head green cabbage (about ½ lb.)

3 celery ribs

1 cucumber

1 cup firmly packed spinach leaves

2 apples

2 celery sprigs for garnish (optional)

Serves 2
Prep time: less than 10 minutes
Each serving: 134 calories 9 calories from fat 1 g fat 0 g saturated fat 4 g protein 33 g carbohydrates

1. Rinse cabbage, trim stem end, and cut into 2-inch cubes. Rinse celery and cut into 2-inch lengths. Rinse cucumber and cut into 2-inch lengths. Rinse spinach. Rinse apples and cut into sixths.

2. Push cabbage, celery, cucumber, spinach, and apples through the juicer, and process until juiced. Stir well and pour juice into two glasses.

3. Serve immediately, garnished with celery sprigs if desired.

Variation: To pulp this recipe in a blender or food processor fitted with a steel blade, core apple and cut all ingredients into pieces no larger than 1 inch.

Juicy Jive

There's no reason to cut up additional fruit or vegetables as a garnish. Just save out a few wedges before pushing the remainder through the juicer. You'll eat the garnish, so the nutritional analysis will hold true. This is true for any fruit or vegetable garnish, but it's not the case for herbs because holding them back will change the delicious taste of the juice.

Cole Slaw and Cauliflower

¼ head green cabbage (about ½ lb.)

2 carrots

1 red bell pepper

4 scallions

1 cup green seedless grapes

2 red bell pepper slices for garnish (optional)

Serves 2

Prep time:
less than 10 minutes

Each serving:
135 calories
9 calories from fat
1 g fat
0 g saturated fat
4 g protein
33 g carbohydrates

1. Rinse cabbage, trim stem end, and cut into 2-inch cubes. Scrub carrots, discard green tops, and cut into 2-inch lengths. Discard cap and seeds from red pepper, and cut into 2-inch pieces. Rinse scallions and cut into 2-inch lengths. Rinse grapes.

2. Push cabbage, carrots, red pepper, scallions, and grapes through the juicer, and process until juiced. Stir well and pour juice into two glasses.

3. Serve immediately, garnished with red pepper slices, if desired.

Variation: To pulp this recipe in a blender or food processor fitted with a steel blade, trim scallions and cut all ingredients into pieces no larger than 1 inch.

Juicy Jive _____

For general cooking, you should discard the ribs as well as the seeds from bell peppers, but that's not necessary when the result is a juice or pulp. The ribs will purée with the rest of the flesh, but the seeds will not, so clean them out of the pepper.

Cabbage, Broccoli, and Orange

¼ head green cabbage (about ½ lb.)

2 broccoli stalks

2 oranges

1 cup firmly packed lettuce leaves

2 broccoli florets for garnish (optional)

Serves 2
Prep time: less than 10 minutes
Each serving: 129 calories 9 calories from fat 1 g fat 0 g saturated fat 7 g protein 29 g carbohydrates

1. Rinse cabbage, trim stem end, and cut into 2-inch cubes. Rinse broccoli and cut into 2-inch cubes. Peel and quarter oranges. Rinse lettuce and cut into 2-inch pieces.

2. Push cabbage, broccoli, oranges, and lettuce through the juicer, and process until juiced. Stir well and pour juice into two glasses.

3. Serve immediately, garnished with broccoli florets, if desired.

Variation: To pulp this recipe in a blender or food processor fitted with a steel blade, peel broccoli stalks, remove seeds from oranges, and cut all ingredients into pieces no larger than 1 inch.

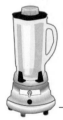

Wrong Spin! _____

Be careful when you're selecting broccoli. While the crowns can look lush and full, if the stems are woody, contain holes, and are cracked, the stalk is old, so pick another one.

Cauliflower and Collards

½ head cauliflower

2 cups firmly packed collard greens

2 cups firmly packed lettuce leaves

1 parsnip

1 apple

2 garlic cloves

2 (2-inch) segments collard greens for garnish (optional)

Serves 2
Prep time: less than 10 minutes
Each serving: 175 calories 9 calories from fat 1 g fat 0 g saturated fat 9 g protein 35 g carbohydrates

1. Rinse cauliflower, trim stem end, discard green leaves, and cut into 2-inch cubes. Rinse collard greens and lettuce and cut into 2-inch lengths. Scrub parsnip, discard green tops, and cut into 2-inch lengths. Rinse apple and cut into sixths. Rinse garlic cloves.

2. Push cauliflower, collard greens, lettuce, parsnip, apple, and garlic through the juicer, and process until juiced. Stir well and pour juice into two glasses.

3. Serve immediately, garnished with sprigs of collard greens if desired.

Variation: To pulp this recipe in a blender or food processor fitted with a steel blade, core apple, peel garlic, and cut all ingredients into pieces no larger than 1 inch.

Pulp Tidbits

Collard greens, or collards, are part of the genre of African-American cooking dubbed "Soul Food." While the dishes themselves are centuries old, the term only came to be used in the mid-twentieth century for food that satisfied the soul. Collards were an important food for gaining iron because the traditional African-American diet was so low in red meats.

Broccoli and Cauliflower

½ head cauliflower

2 broccoli stalks

2 celery ribs

2 apples

2 cauliflower florets for garnish (optional)

Serves 2
Prep time:
less than 10 minutes
Each serving:
149 calories
9 calories from fat
1 g fat
0 g saturated fat
9 g protein
33 g carbohydrates

1. Rinse cauliflower, trim stem, discard green leaves, and cut into 2-inch cubes. Rinse broccoli and celery, and cut into 2-inch lengths. Rinse apples and cut into sixths.

2. Push cauliflower, broccoli, celery, and apples through the juicer, and process until juiced. Stir well and pour juice into two glasses.

3. Serve immediately, garnished with cauliflower florets if desired.

Variation: To pulp this recipe in a blender or food processor fitted with a steel blade, peel broccoli stalks, core apples, and cut all ingredients into pieces no larger than 1 inch.

Juicy Jive

You'll see broccoli rabe—sometimes dubbed rapini, which is the Italian name—in many supermarkets. The flavor is more intense than that of common broccoli, but feel free to substitute it in any juice recipe. You'll use the same weight as conventional broccoli because the stalks are much thinner.

Asian Broccoli

4 broccoli stalks

4 scallions

3 celery ribs

2 garlic cloves

3 TB. sliced ginger

1 TB. tamari

2 celery sprigs for garnish (optional)

Serves 2
Prep time:
less than 10 minutes
Each serving:
102 calories
9 calories from fat
1 g fat
0 g saturated fat
9 g protein
20 g carbohydrates

1. Rinse broccoli, scallions, celery, and garlic cloves. Cut into 2-inch lengths.

2. Push broccoli, scallions, celery, garlic, and ginger through the juicer, and process until juiced. Pour juice into two glasses, and add ½ tablespoon *tamari* to each. Stir well.

3. Serve immediately, garnished with celery sprigs if desired.

Variation: To pulp this recipe in a blender or food processor fitted with a steel blade, peel broccoli stalks, trim scallions, peel garlic and ginger, and cut all ingredients into pieces no larger than 1 inch.

Liquid Lingo

Tamari, like soy sauce, is made from soybeans. But its flavor is more mellow and less salty, and its texture is thicker than soy sauce. It's a common ingredient found in the Asian section of most supermarkets.

Broccoli, Red Pepper, and Cucumber

3 broccoli stalks

1 red bell pepper

$^{1}/_{2}$ cucumber

2 scallions

1 orange

$^{1}/_{4}$ tsp. cayenne

2 cucumber spears for garnish (optional)

Serves 2
Prep time: less than 10 minutes
Each serving: 113 calories 9 calories from fat 1 g fat 0 g saturated fat 7 g protein 25 g carbohydrates

1. Rinse broccoli and cut into 2-inch lengths. Rinse red pepper and discard cap and seeds. Rinse cucumber and scallions, and cut into 2-inch lengths. Peel and quarter orange.

2. Push broccoli, bell pepper, cucumber, scallions, and orange through the juicer, and process until juiced. Pour juice into two glasses, and stir $^{1}/_{8}$ teaspoon cayenne into each glass.

3. Serve immediately, garnished with cucumber spears if desired.

Variation: To pulp this recipe in a blender or food processor fitted with a steel blade, peel broccoli stalks, trim scallions, and cut all ingredients into pieces no larger than 1 inch.

Juicy Jive

If you've ever wondered why red bell peppers are always more expensive than green, it's because they are the same peppers, but they've been left on the plant to mature. That's why they're sweeter and less acidic than green peppers. But they are also more perishable to ship, which accounts for their premium price.

Broccoli and Kale

2 broccoli stalks

3 celery ribs

1 cup firmly packed kale leaves

¼ cup firmly packed parsley sprigs

1 apple

2 celery sprigs for garnish (optional)

Serves 2

Prep time:
less than 10 minutes

Each serving:
98 calories
9 calories from fat
1 g fat
0 g saturated fat
5 g protein
22 g carbohydrates

1. Rinse broccoli, celery, and *kale*, and cut into 2-inch lengths. Rinse parsley. Rinse apple and cut into sixths.

2. Push broccoli, celery, kale, parsley, and apple through the juicer, and process until juiced. Stir well and pour juice into two glasses.

3. Serve immediately, garnished with celery sprigs if desired.

Variation: To pulp this recipe in a blender or food processor fitted with a steel blade, peel broccoli stalks, core apple, and cut all ingredients into pieces no larger than 1 inch.

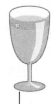

Liquid Lingo

Kale is the renegade cousin of the cabbage family. Its flavor is very mild, and it has frilly deep green leaves that look like a bouquet of flowers rather than a tight head. Buy small heads that are perky and not limp.

Brussels Sprout and Lemon

2 pints Brussels sprouts

3 celery ribs

2 apples

1 carrot

¼ lemon

¼ cup firmly packed parsley sprigs

2 parsley sprigs for garnish (optional)

Serves 2
Prep time: less than 10 minutes
Each serving: 174 calories 9 calories from fat 1 g fat 0 g saturated fat 7 g protein 41 g carbohydrates

1. Rinse Brussels sprouts, trim stem ends, and discard any discolored leaves. Rinse celery and cut into 2-inch lengths. Rinse apples and cut into sixths. Scrub carrot, discard green tops, and cut into 2-inch lengths. Peel lemon. Rinse parsley.

2. Push Brussels sprouts, celery, apples, carrot, lemon, and parsley through the juicer, and process until juiced. Stir well and pour juice into two glasses.

3. Serve immediately, garnished with parsley sprigs if desired.

Variation: To pulp this recipe in a blender or food processor fitted with a steel blade, core apple, remove seeds from lemon, and cut all ingredients into pieces no larger than 1 inch.

Pulp Tidbits

Brussels sprouts are so named because they were first cultivated in Belgium in the sixteenth century. Unlike their cabbage cousins, these tiny heads grow in many rows on a single long stem. In the fall when they're in season, it's possible to purchase them this way in some markets.

Chapter 7

Our Good Friend Herb

In This Chapter

◆ Vegetable and herb combinations

◆ Creamy juices

◆ Spicy treats

Fresh herbs are like the frosting on a cake. They play their own role, but they bring the whole thing together. You probably know this from cooking with herbs, and the recipes in this chapter will show you that the same synergy occurs when you add herbs to juices.

When put through the juicer, the flavor of fresh herbs remains subtle. They will take on a stronger flavor if the drink is pulped in a blender or food processor.

While you add herbs for flavor rather than nutritional benefits, over the centuries herbs have been used as cures for everything from indigestion to migraines and also as aromatic teas.

Handle with Care

Fresh herbs are very perishable, especially if they've come from supermarkets that mist them with water on a regular basis. This watering basically causes them to rot.

Wrap herbs with woody stems, such as rosemary and thyme, in a damp paper towel and place them inside a heavy plastic bag.

A large group of herbs have tender stems. This group includes basil, cilantro, dill, mint, oregano, parsley, and tarragon. Treat these herbs like a bouquet of flowers. Trim the stem ends, and place the herbs with the stems into a deep glass. Add enough water to come one inch up the stems, and then wrap the glass in a plastic bag. Stand it upright in the refrigerator, and the water should preserve the freshness of the herbs for up to five days.

Dilled Cucumber

3 cucumbers

2 scallions

⅓ cup firmly packed dill weed

1 cup plain nonfat yogurt

Salt and freshly ground black pepper to taste

2 dill sprigs for garnish (optional)

Serves 2
Prep time: less than 10 minutes
Each serving: 142 calories 9 calories from fat 1 g fat 0 g saturated fat 10 g protein 27 g carbohydrates

1. Rinse cucumbers and scallions, and cut into 2-inch lengths. Rinse dill.

2. Push cucumbers, scallions, and dill through the juicer, and process until juiced. Pour juice into a blender and add yogurt. Blend for 30 seconds, and pour juice into two glasses. Season each glass to taste with salt and pepper.

3. Serve immediately, garnished with dill sprigs if desired.

Variation: To pulp this recipe in a blender or food processor fitted with a steel blade, trim scallions and cut all ingredients into pieces no larger than 1 inch. If using a blender or food processor, add yogurt along with other ingredients.

Pulp Tidbits

Acidophilus, an ingredient used to thicken yogurt, is a friendly bacteria, called a "probiotic" in some natural food circles. It lives in the intestines and helps prevent intestinal infections. Taking antibiotics can disturb the body's balance of friendly bacteria, which is why eating yogurt when taking antibiotics is frequently recommended.

Green Pepper and Rosemary

3 green bell peppers

1 cup green seedless grapes

2 celery ribs

3 sprigs rosemary

2 rosemary sprigs for garnish (optional)

Serves 2
Prep time: less than 10 minutes
Each serving: 101 calories 9 calories from fat 1 g fat 3 g protein 25 g carbohydrates

1. Discard cap and seeds from peppers, and cut into 2-inch pieces. Rinse grapes. Rinse celery and cut into 2-inch lengths. Rinse rosemary and remove leaves from stems if stems are woody.

2. Push peppers, grapes, celery, and rosemary through the juicer, and process until juiced. Stir well, and pour juice into two glasses.

3. Serve immediately, garnished with rosemary sprigs if desired.

Variation: To pulp this recipe in a blender or food processor fitted with a steel blade, cut all ingredients into pieces no larger than 1 inch.

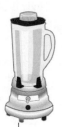

Wrong Spin! _____

Rosemary is an herb that has many different species. Some of them have soft, supple stems like those of parsley or oregano. And some are so woody they are even sold as skewers! If you have soft stems, push them through the juicer, but if the stems are woody, pull the leaves off them.

Tomato and Basil

6 tomatoes

1 cup firmly packed basil leaves

¼ lemon

2 garlic cloves

2 scallions

Salt and freshly ground black pepper to taste

2 basil sprigs for garnish (optional)

Serves 2
Prep time: less than 10 minutes
Each serving: 85 calories 9 calories from fat 1 g fat 0 g saturated fat 4 g protein 19 g carbohydrates

1. Rinse tomatoes and cut into quarters. Rinse basil. Peel lemon. Rinse garlic cloves and scallions.

2. Push tomatoes, basil, lemon, garlic, and scallions through the juicer, and process until juiced. Stir well and pour juice into two glasses. Season each glass to taste with salt and pepper.

3. Serve immediately, garnished with basil sprigs if desired.

Variation: To pulp this recipe in a blender or food processor fitted with a steel blade, core tomatoes, remove seeds from lemon, peel garlic, trim scallions, and cut all ingredients into pieces no larger than 1 inch.

Pulp Tidbits

Basil has been used in the kitchen since as early as 400 B.C.E. when Greek botanist Chrysippos described it as one of his favorite seasonings. The Romans used it in their bouquet garni, and the Byzantines used it to flavor sauces.

Zucchini, Tomato, and Oregano

4 medium zucchini

3 tomatoes

2 celery ribs

2 scallions

2 garlic cloves

¼ cup firmly packed oregano leaves

Salt and freshly ground black pepper to taste

2 oregano sprigs for garnish (optional)

Serves 2
Prep time: less than 10 minutes
Each serving: 123 calories 18 calories from fat 2 g fat 0 g saturated fat 7 g protein 26 g carbohydrates

1. Rinse zucchini, trim caps and cut into 2-inch lengths. Rinse tomatoes and cut into quarters. Rinse celery and scallions, and cut into 2-inch lengths. Rinse garlic cloves. Rinse oregano and remove leaves from stems if stems are woody.

2. Push zucchini, tomatoes, celery, scallions, garlic, and oregano through the juicer, and process until juiced. Pour juice into two glasses. Season each glass to taste with salt and pepper and stir well.

3. Serve immediately, garnished with oregano sprigs if desired.

Variation: To pulp this recipe in a blender or food processor fitted with a steel blade, core tomatoes, trim scallions, peel garlic, remove oregano leaves from stems, and cut all ingredients into pieces no larger than 1 inch.

Juicy Jive

Oregano is one of the herbs that works very well as a raw ingredient for salads. Rinse the sprigs, pull the leaves off the stems, and add them to mixed salad greens. They will add a peppery richness.

Celery and Tarragon

8 celery ribs

2 scallions

¼ cup firmly packed tarragon sprigs

⅔ cup plain nonfat yogurt

Salt and freshly ground black pepper to taste

2 tarragon sprigs for garnish (optional)

Serves 2

Prep time:
less than 10 minutes

Each serving:
106 calories
9 calories from fat
1 g fat
0 g saturated fat
9 g protein
18 g carbohydrates

1. Rinse celery and scallions, and cut into 2-inch lengths. Rinse tarragon, and remove leaves from stems if stems are woody.

2. Push celery, scallions, and tarragon through the juicer, and process until juiced. Pour juice into a blender and add yogurt. Blend for 30 seconds, and pour juice into two glasses. Season each glass to taste with salt and pepper and stir well.

3. Serve immediately, garnished with tarragon sprigs if desired.

Variation: To pulp this recipe in a blender or food processor fitted with a steel blade, trim scallions, remove tarragon leaves from stems, and cut all ingredients into pieces no larger than 1 inch. If using a blender or food processor, add yogurt along with other ingredients.

Pulp Tidbits

Nomadic tribes in the Balkans are thought to have started yogurt-making thousands of years ago, and yogurt is still used extensively in dishes springing from that region. The process probably started by accident, but then the tribesmen realized that it preserved the freshness of milk.

Southwest Tomato

6 tomatoes

1 red bell pepper

¼ red onion

1 jalapeño chili

⅓ cup firmly packed cilantro sprigs

2 garlic cloves

Salt and cayenne to taste

2 cilantro sprigs for garnish (optional)

Serves 2
Prep time: less than 10 minutes
Each serving: 109 calories 18 calories from fat 2 g fat 0 g saturated fat 4 g protein 24 g carbohydrates

1. Rinse tomatoes and quarter them. Rinse bell pepper, and discard cap and seeds. Peel onion and cut into 2-inch cubes. Rinse jalapeño and discard cap and seeds. Rinse cilantro and garlic.

2. Push tomatoes, bell pepper, onion, jalapeño, cilantro, and garlic through the juicer, and process until juiced. Pour juice into two glasses. Season each glass to taste with salt and pepper and stir well.

3. Serve immediately, garnished with cilantro sprigs if desired.

Variation: To pulp this recipe in a blender or food processor fitted with a steel blade, core tomatoes, peel garlic, and cut all ingredients into pieces no larger than 1 inch.

Juicy Jive

Cilantro is not at the top of the Hit Parade for many people, and if you're among them, the best substitute at all times is Italian flat leaf parsley. You'll still get a fresh taste without the pungency.

Provençale Tomato and Red Pepper

3 tomatoes

2 red bell peppers

½ cucumber

2 garlic cloves

¼ cup firmly packed parsley sprigs

2 sprigs thyme

1 sprig rosemary

Salt and freshly ground black pepper to taste

2 rosemary sprigs for garnish (optional)

Serves 2
Prep time: less than 10 minutes
Each serving: 94 calories 9 calories from fat 1 g fat 0 g saturated fat 4 g protein 21 g carbohydrates

1. Rinse tomatoes and cut into quarters. Rinse bell peppers, discard caps and seeds, and cut into 2-inch pieces. Rinse cucumber and cut into 2-inch lengths. Rinse garlic cloves and parsley. Rinse thyme and rosemary, and remove leaves from the stems if stems are woody.

2. Push tomatoes, bell peppers, cucumber, garlic, parsley, thyme, and rosemary through the juicer, and process until juiced. Pour juice into two glasses. Season each glass to taste with salt and pepper and stir well.

3. Serve immediately, garnished with rosemary sprigs if desired.

Variation: To pulp this recipe in a blender or food processor fitted with a steel blade, core tomatoes, peel garlic, remove thyme and rosemary leaves from stems, and cut all ingredients into pieces no larger than 1 inch.

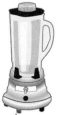

Wrong Spin!

Herbs have a tendency to be full of grit and sand. Keep in mind they grow close to the ground. So if a bunch looks dirty, let the sprigs soak in a bowl of ice water for a few minutes, and then remove them from the top. Don't place them into a colander or the grit will go right back onto the herbs.

Cucumber and Cilantro

3 cucumbers

⅓ cup firmly packed cilantro sprigs

1 jalapeño or serrano chili

½ cup plain nonfat yogurt

½ cup pine nuts

Salt and freshly ground black pepper to taste

2 cilantro sprigs for garnish (optional)

Serves 2

Prep time:
less than 10 minutes

Each serving:
338 calories
216 calories from fat
24 g fat
2 g saturated fat
11 g protein
26 g carbohydrates

1. Rinse cucumbers and cut into 2-inch lengths. Rinse cilantro. Rinse jalapeño and discard cap and seeds.

2. Push cucumbers, cilantro, and jalapeño through the juicer, and process until juiced. Pour juice into a blender, and add yogurt and *pine nuts.* Blend for 30 seconds, and pour juice into two glasses. Season each glass to taste with salt and pepper.

3. Serve immediately, garnished with cilantro sprigs if desired.

Variation: To pulp this recipe in a blender or food processor fitted with a steel blade, cut all ingredients into pieces no larger than 1-inch. If using a blender or food processor, add yogurt and pine nuts along with other ingredients.

Liquid Lingo

Pine nuts, also called *piñon* in Spanish and *pignoli* in Italian, are the nuts located inside the pine cones of various species of evergreen. To remove them, you must heat the pine cones and then pull the nuts, which are in thin shells, out by hand. This labor-intensive method is why they are so expensive.

Minted Pea and Cucumber

3 cups peas

2 cucumbers

2 celery ribs

2 scallions

¼ cup firmly packed mint sprigs

2 mint sprigs for garnish (optional)

Serves 2
Prep time: less than 10 minutes
Each serving: 234 calories 9 calories from fat 1 g fat 0 g saturated fat 14 g protein 45 g carbohydrates

1. Rinse peas. Rinse cucumbers, celery, and scallions, and cut into 2-inch lengths.

2. Push peas, cucumbers, celery, scallions, and mint through the juicer, and process until juiced. Stir well and pour juice into two glasses.

3. Serve immediately, garnished with mint sprigs if desired.

Variation: To pulp this recipe in a blender or food processor fitted with a steel blade, trim scallions and cut all ingredients into pieces no larger than 1 inch.

Pulp Tidbits

In Greek mythology, mint was once a nymph named Mentha. Because she angered Persephone, Pluto's wife, she turned her into this aromatic herb as permanent revenge.

Potato and Chive

2 large red potatoes

2 parsnips

2 celery ribs

$\frac{1}{3}$ cup firmly packed chives

1 cup plain nonfat yogurt

Salt and freshly ground black pepper to taste

2 celery sprigs for garnish (optional)

Serves 2
Prep time: less than 10 minutes
Each serving: 335 calories 9 calories from fat 1 g fat 0 g saturated fat 13.5 g protein 71 g carbohydrates

1. Scrub potatoes well, and cut into 2-inch cubes. Scrub parsnips, discard tops, and cut into 2-inch lengths. Rinse celery and chives, and cut into 2-inch lengths.

2. Push potatoes, parsnips, celery, and chives through the juicer, and process until juiced. Pour juice into a blender and add yogurt. Blend for 30 seconds, and pour juice into two glasses. Season each glass to taste with salt and pepper.

3. Serve immediately, garnished with celery sprigs if desired.

Variation: To pulp this recipe in a blender or food processor fitted with a steel blade, cut all ingredients into pieces no larger than 1 inch. If using a blender or food processor, add yogurt along with other ingredients.

Juicy Jive

If you don't have any chives, the best substitute in this or any recipe is the finely sliced green tops of scallions. They have the same mild onion flavor.

Chapter 8

Soups to Slurp

In This Chapter

- ◆ Juice versions of popular cold soups
- ◆ Creamy juices made with healthful yogurt
- ◆ Spicy juices to wake up your taste buds

What makes the recipes in this chapter different from others in the vegetable part of this book is that they're all based on cold soups. And if you choose to pulp them rather than juice them, you can easily serve them as soups.

Most of these juices are enlivened with ingredients to boost the flavor. Some contain various forms of vinegar, while others have some spices added at the end. What you'll find is that the flavors are complex and perk the palate.

Chilled to Perfection

The temperature of almost all the juices in this book is a matter of personal preference. I prefer fruit juices at room temperature because I think the aroma of fresh fruits is strongest when it's warm, but I prefer most vegetable juices chilled.

I have formulated the recipes in this chapter with all the ingredients well chilled. So allow yourself some time for that step.

Carrot Gazpacho

4 carrots

4 scallions

4 ripe plum tomatoes

2 celery ribs

½ cucumber

½ red bell pepper

1 lime

Cayenne to taste

2 cucumber slices for garnish (optional)

Serves 2
Prep time: less than 10 minutes
Each serving: 147 calories 9 calories from fat 1 g fat 0 g saturated fat 5 g protein 35 g carbohydrates

1. Scrub carrots, discard green tops, and cut into 2-inch lengths. Rinse scallions and cut into 2-inch lengths. Rinse and quarter tomatoes. Rinse celery and cucumber, and cut into 2-inch lengths. Rinse bell pepper, discard cap and seeds, and cut into 2-inch pieces. Peel lime.

2. Push carrots, scallions, tomatoes, celery, cucumber, bell pepper, and lime through the juicer, and process until juiced. Pour juice into two glasses, season each glass to taste with *cayenne*, and stir well.

3. Serve immediately, garnished with cucumber slices if desired.

Variation: To pulp this recipe in a blender or food processor fitted with a steel blade, trim scallions, core tomatoes, and cut all ingredients into pieces no larger than 1 inch.

Liquid Lingo

Cayenne is not actually a pepper because it doesn't come from peppercorns. This pungent, spicy powder that originated in French Guyana is made from ground cayenne chili peppers. In supermarkets it's sometimes just called red pepper.

Gazpacho

4 ripe beefsteak tomatoes

1 cucumber

1 red bell pepper

1 jalapeño chili

½ small red onion

3 garlic cloves

¼ cup firmly packed cilantro sprigs

¼ cup balsamic vinegar

Salt and freshly ground black pepper to taste

2 cilantro sprigs for garnish (optional)

Serves 2
Prep time:
less than 10 minutes
Each serving:
193 calories
18 calories from fat
2 g fat
0 g saturated fat
6 g protein
43 g carbohydrates

1. Rinse and quarter tomatoes. Rinse cucumber and cut into 2-inch lengths. Discard cap and seeds from bell pepper and jalapeño, and cut into slices. Peel onion. Rinse garlic and cilantro.

2. Push tomatoes, cucumber, red bell pepper, jalapeño, onion, garlic, and cilantro through the juicer, and process until juiced. Pour juice into two glasses, stir ⅛ cup balsamic vinegar into each glass, and season each glass to taste with salt and pepper.

3. Serve immediately, garnished with cilantro sprigs if desired.

Variation: To pulp this recipe in a blender or food processor fitted with a steel blade, core tomatoes, peel garlic, and cut all ingredients into pieces no larger than 1 inch.

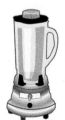

Wrong Spin! _____

Heady and rich-tasting balsamic vinegar is made from Trebbiano grapes and gets its sweetness from long aging. But be careful when purchasing it, because many of the less expensive vinegars contain sulfites that are added to inhibit the growth of bacteria.

Carrot and Spinach Gazpacho

4 ripe beefsteak tomatoes

4 scallions

2 carrots

2 celery ribs

1 cup firmly packed spinach leaves

1 cucumber

2 garlic cloves

¼ cup white wine vinegar

Salt and freshly ground black pepper to taste

2 carrot sticks for garnish (optional)

Serves 2

Prep time:
less than 10 minutes

Each serving:
135 calories
9 calories from fat
1 g fat
0 g saturated fat
5 g protein
28 g carbohydrates

1. Rinse tomatoes and cut into quarters. Rinse scallions and cut into 2-inch lengths. Scrub carrots, discard tops, and cut into 2-inch lengths. Rinse celery and cut into 2-inch lengths. Rinse spinach. Rinse cucumber and cut into 2-inch lengths. Rinse garlic cloves.

2. Push tomatoes, scallions, carrots, celery, spinach, cucumber, and garlic through the juicer, and process until juiced. Pour juice into two glasses, stir ⅛ cup vinegar into each glass, and season each glass to taste with salt and pepper.

3. Serve immediately, garnished with carrot sticks if desired.

Variation: To pulp this recipe in a blender or food processor fitted with a steel blade, core tomatoes, trim scallions, peel garlic, and cut all ingredients into pieces no larger than 1 inch.

Pulp Tidbits

The prototype for all the soups we now dub gazpacho comes from the Andalusia region in southern Spain. The original soup was made with tomatoes as the base and enlivened with other vegetables, but today it's really any uncooked vegetable soup that includes garlic, some sort of acid, and at least a few tomatoes.

Creamy Avocado

4 ripe plum tomatoes

1 Anaheim pepper

1 cucumber

½ small red onion

½ lime

¼ cup firmly packed cilantro sprigs

2 garlic cloves

2 avocadoes

½ cup plain nonfat yogurt

Salt and freshly ground black pepper to taste

2 cilantro sprigs for garnish (optional)

Serves 2
Prep time: less than 10 minutes
Each serving: 425 calories 243 calories from fat 27 g fat 4 g saturated fat 11 g protein 44 g carbohydrates

1. Rinse and quarter tomatoes. Discard cap and seeds of *Anaheim pepper*. Rinse cucumber and cut into 2-inch lengths. Peel red onion. Peel lime. Rinse cilantro sprigs and garlic cloves. Peel avocadoes, discard seeds, and cut into 1-inch pieces.

2. Push tomatoes, Anaheim pepper, cucumber, onion, lime, cilantro, and garlic through the juicer, and process until juiced. Pour juice into a blender, and add avocadoes and yogurt. Blend for 30 seconds, and pour juice into two glasses. Season each glass to taste with salt and pepper.

3. Serve immediately, garnished with cilantro sprigs if desired.

Variation: To pulp this recipe in a blender or food processor fitted with a steel blade, core tomatoes, remove seeds from lime, peel garlic, and cut all ingredients into pieces no larger than 1 inch. If using a blender or food processor, add avocado and yogurt along with other ingredients.

Liquid Lingo

Anaheim peppers are named for the city in California made famous by Disneyland, and they're light green in color and have a long narrow shape. They have a basically sweet taste with just a hint of a bite, so they're used frequently for stuffing as *chilis rellaños*, and they're the species of pepper canned as mild green chilies.

Borscht

2 large beets

2 oranges

1 cucumber

3 scallions

1 cup plain nonfat yogurt

2 cucumber spears for garnish (optional)

Serves 2
Prep time: less than 10 minutes
Each serving: 196 calories 9 calories from fat 1 g fat 0 g saturated fat 11 g protein 40 g carbohydrates

1. Scrub beets well, discard tops if wilted but rinse and use if not, and cut into 2-inch cubes. Peel and quarter oranges. Rinse cucumber and cut into 2-inch lengths. Rinse scallions.

2. Push beets, oranges, cucumber, and scallions through the juicer, and process until juiced. Pour juice into a blender and add yogurt. Blend for 30 seconds, and pour juice into two glasses.

3. Serve immediately, garnished with cucumber spears if desired.

Variation: To pulp this recipe in a blender or food processor fitted with a steel blade, remove seeds from oranges, trim scallions, and cut all ingredients into pieces no larger than 1 inch. If using a blender or food processor, add yogurt along with other ingredients.

Pulp Tidbits

Borscht, always made with beets and sometimes made with meat, is of Russian and Polish origin. It was popular with the Jews who emigrated from those countries, and during the 1930s, resorts in New York's Catskill Mountains that featured Jewish entertainers became known as the "Borscht Belt."

Spiced Carrot and Cauliflower

$\frac{1}{2}$ head cauliflower

3 carrots

1 cup firmly packed spinach leaves

4 TB. sliced ginger

$\frac{1}{2}$ tsp. ground cinnamon

Cayenne to taste

2 carrot sticks for garnish (optional)

Serves 2
Prep time: less than 10 minutes
Each serving: 91 calories 9 calories from fat 1 g fat 0 g saturated fat 6 g protein 18 g carbohydrates

1. Rinse cauliflower, trim stem end, discard green leaves, and cut into 2-inch cubes. Scrub carrots, discard tops, and cut into 2-inch lengths. Rinse spinach.

2. Push cauliflower, carrots, spinach, and ginger through the juicer, and process until juiced. Pour juice into two glasses, and stir $\frac{1}{4}$ teaspoon cinnamon and cayenne to taste into each glass.

3. Serve immediately, garnished with carrot sticks if desired.

Variation: To pulp this recipe in a blender or food processor fitted with a steel blade, peel ginger and cut all ingredients into pieces no larger than 1 inch. If using a blender or food processor, add cinnamon and cayenne along with other ingredients.

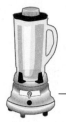

Wrong Spin!

You might think it's wasteful to discard the cauliflower leaves, but it's not. Their very strong taste would overwhelm the juice.

Southwest Celery

8 celery ribs

1 fennel bulb

3 scallions

1 jalapeño chili

2 garlic cloves

¼ cup firmly packed cilantro sprigs

½ tsp. ground cumin

2 cilantro sprigs for garnish (optional)

Serves 2
Prep time:
less than 10 minutes
Each serving:
77 calories
9 calories from fat
1 g fat
0 g saturated fat
4 g protein
17 g carbohydrates

1. Rinse celery and cut into 2-inch lengths. Rinse fennel bulb, trim off stem end, and cut into 2-inch cubes. Rinse scallions. Discard cap and seeds of jalapeño. Rinse garlic and cilantro.

2. Push celery, fennel, scallions, jalapeño, garlic, and cilantro through the juicer, and process until juiced. Pour juice into two glasses, and stir ¼ teaspoon *cumin* into each glass.

3. Serve immediately, garnished with cilantro sprigs if desired.

Variation: To pulp this recipe in a blender or food processor fitted with a steel blade, trim scallions, peel garlic, and cut all ingredients into pieces no larger than 1 inch. If using a blender or food processor, add cumin along with other ingredients.

Liquid Lingo

Cumin is frequently found in markets under its Spanish name, comino. The seeds from which it's ground are the dried fruit from a plant in the parsley family, which is very aromatic. It's one of the major ingredients in commercial chili powder, so you can always substitute chili powder if necessary.

Mixed Pepper

2 red bell peppers

2 orange bell peppers

1 cucumber

1 fennel bulb

Freshly ground black pepper to taste

2 pepper slices for garnish (optional)

Serves 2
Prep time:
less than 10 minutes
Each serving:
123 calories
9 calories from fat
1 g fat
0 g saturated fat
5 g protein
29 g carbohydrates

1. Rinse red and orange bell peppers, discard caps and seeds, and cut into 2-inch pieces. Rinse cucumber and cut into 2-inch lengths. Rinse fennel bulb, trim off stem end, and cut into 2-inch cubes.

2. Push bell peppers, cucumber, and fennel through the juicer, and process until juiced. Pour juice into two glasses, season each glass to taste with pepper, and stir well.

3. Serve immediately, garnished with pepper slices if desired.

Variation: To pulp this recipe in a blender or food processor fitted with a steel blade, cut all ingredients into pieces no larger than 1 inch.

Juicy Jive

You can use all peppers of the same color or vary the recipe by using yellow instead of the ones listed, but don't use green peppers even though they're always lower in price. They are bitter by comparison to more mature colored peppers, all of which are green and bitter in their immature form.

Curried Carrot

4 carrots

3 apples

2 celery ribs

2 garlic cloves

2 scallions

1 tsp. curry powder

2 celery sprigs for garnish (optional)

Serves 2
Prep time: less than 10 minutes
Each serving: 179 calories 9 calories from fat 1 g fat 0 g saturated fat 3 g protein 45 g carbohydrates

1. Scrub carrots, discard tops, and cut into 2-inch lengths. Rinse apples and cut into sixths. Rinse celery and cut into 2-inch lengths. Rinse garlic cloves and scallions.

2. Push carrots, apples, celery, garlic cloves, and scallions through the juicer, and process until juiced. Pour juice into two glasses, and stir ½ teaspoon curry powder into each glass.

3. Serve immediately, garnished with celery sprigs if desired.

Variation: To pulp this recipe in a blender or food processor fitted with a steel blade, core apples, peel garlic, trim scallions, and cut all ingredients into pieces no larger than 1 inch. If using a blender or food processor, add curry powder along with other ingredients.

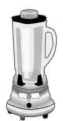

Wrong Spin!

While it's a good idea to toss out any dried herb or spice that's been opened for more than six months, abbreviate the life of curry powder to two months. This ground blend, made from up to 20 herbs and spices, loses its flavor and aroma very quickly.

Asian Tomato

6 ripe plum tomatoes

2 celery ribs

3 scallions

2 garlic cloves

2 TB. sliced ginger

1 TB. tamari

2 celery sprigs for garnish (optional)

Serves 2
Prep time:
less than 10 minutes
Each serving:
108 calories
9 calories from fat
1 g fat
0 g saturated fat
5 g protein
23 g carbohydrates

1. Rinse tomatoes and cut into quarters. Rinse celery and cut into 2-inch lengths. Rinse scallions and cut into 2-inch lengths. Rinse garlic cloves.

2. Push tomatoes, celery, scallions, garlic, and ginger through the juicer, and process until juiced. Pour juice into two glasses, divide tamari between the two, and stir well.

3. Serve immediately, garnished with celery sprigs if desired.

Variation: To pulp this recipe in a blender or food processor fitted with a steel blade, core tomatoes, trim scallions, peel garlic and ginger, and cut all ingredients into pieces no larger than 1 inch. If using a blender or food processor, add tamari along with other ingredients.

Juicy Jive _____

If you're worried about sodium in your diet, then substitute reduced-sodium soy sauce for the tamari in this or any recipe. It will add a similar flavor with less sodium.

Pea and Carrot

2 cups fresh peas

3 carrots

2 parsnips

1 apple

½ medium onion

½ fennel bulb

¼ cup firmly packed parsley sprigs

2 parsley sprigs for garnish (optional)

Serves 2
Prep time: less than 10 minutes
Each serving: 375 calories 18 calories from fat 2 g fat 0 g saturated fat 13 g protein 83 g carbohydrates

1. Rinse peas. Scrub carrots and parsnips, discard tops, and cut into 2-inch lengths. Rinse apple and cut into sixths. Peel onion. Rinse fennel bulb, trim stem end, and cut into 2-inch cubes. Rinse parsley.

2. Push peas, carrots, parsnips, apple, onion, fennel, and parsley through the juicer, and process until juiced. Stir well and pour juice into two glasses.

3. Serve immediately, garnished with parsley sprigs if desired.

Variation: To pulp this recipe in a blender or food processor fitted with a steel blade, core apple and cut all ingredients into pieces no larger than 1 inch.

Juicy Jive

While frozen peas are quick and easy to thaw, they are already blanched before they're frozen so some of the nutrients are lost. But in a pinch or when fresh peas are not in season, they are a good substitute. However, all canned vegetables, not just peas, should be avoided.

Chapter 9

Combo Creations

In This Chapter

- ◆ Balancing fruits and vegetables
- ◆ Colorful mixtures with herbs and spices
- ◆ Refreshing thirst quenchers

Many recipes in this book combine vegetables and fruits. But these recipes give them both equal status as the stars of the various juices.

Fruits are inherently sweet, while only vegetables such as carrots, parsnips, and beets can make that claim. At the same time, mild vegetables—such as cucumbers and celery—need some boosting in the flavor department. These qualities produce a complex flavor profile.

A Balancing Act

One of my goals in writing this book is to give you the confidence to start experimenting with different juices so you can increase your repertoire of options and suit your personal taste. This chapter is a good place to begin.

When you're concocting a juice, think about colors as well as flavors. Remember we eat with our eyes before our taste buds enter the picture, so you want a juice to have a pleasing hue.

Then think about the Chinese concept of yin-yang. In this case it means balancing flavors. Sweet should be balanced by sour, and hot should be balanced by mild.

If you keep these precepts in mind when you're making the recipes in this chapter, you're on your way to improvisational juicing!

Minted Honeydew and Celery

¼ honeydew melon

4 celery ribs

3 scallions

1 cucumber

⅓ cup firmly packed mint sprigs

½ cup plain nonfat yogurt

¼ cup white wine vinegar

Salt and freshly ground white pepper to taste

2 mint sprigs for garnish (optional)

Serves 2

Prep time:
less than 10 minutes

Each serving:
135 calories
9 calories from fat
1 g fat
0 g saturated fat
6 g protein
27 g carbohydrates

1. Peel honeydew and cut into 2-inch cubes.

    Rinse celery, scallions, and cucumber, and cut into 2-inch lengths. Rinse mint sprigs.

2. Push melon, celery, scallions, cucumber, and mint through the juicer, and process until juiced. Pour juice into a blender, and add yogurt and vinegar. Blend for 30 seconds; then pour juice into two glasses. Season each glass to taste with salt and pepper.

3. Serve immediately, garnished with mint sprigs if desired.

Variation: To pulp this recipe in a blender or food processor fitted with a steel blade, discard melon seeds, trim scallions, and cut all ingredients into pieces no larger than 1 inch. If using a blender or food processor, add yogurt and vinegar with other ingredients.

Juicy Jive

You can always use soft tofu in place of yogurt or sour cream in a recipe to make it non-dairy. Use the same amount of tofu as the dairy ingredient, and then add 1 tablespoon lemon juice for each cup of yogurt to give the dish the same tangy flavor.

Spicy Cantaloupe and Cucumber

$\frac{1}{2}$ cantaloupe

2 carrots

1 cucumber

4 scallions

1 orange

$\frac{1}{4}$ lemon

$\frac{1}{4}$ cup cider vinegar

Cayenne to taste

2 cantaloupe spears for garnish (optional)

Serves 2
Prep time: less than 10 minutes
Each serving: 164 calories 9 calories from fat 1 g fat 0 g saturated fat 4 g protein 38 g carbohydrates

1. Peel cantaloupe and cut into 2-inch cubes. Scrub carrots, discard tops, and cut into 2-inch lengths. Rinse cucumber and scallions, and cut into 2-inch lengths. Peel and quarter orange. Peel lemon.

2. Push cantaloupe, carrots, cucumber, scallions, orange, and lemon through the juicer, and process until juiced. Pour juice into two glasses, stir $\frac{1}{8}$ cup *cider vinegar* into each glass, and season to taste with cayenne.

3. Serve immediately, garnished with cantaloupe spears if desired.

Variation: To pulp this recipe in a blender or food processor fitted with a steel blade, discard cantaloupe seeds, trim scallions, remove orange and lemon seeds, and cut all ingredients into pieces no larger than 1 inch. If using a blender or food processor, add vinegar and cayenne with other ingredients.

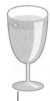

Liquid Lingo

Cider vinegar has an underlying fruity flavor and is made from distilled apple cider. It's milder than wine vinegars or distilled white vinegar, and the best substitute would be half balsamic vinegar mixed with half white wine vinegar.

Gingered Beet and Apple

3 apples

2 beets

1 pear

$^{1}/_{2}$ lemon

4 TB. sliced ginger

2 apple wedges for garnish (optional)

Serves 2

Prep time:
less than 10 minutes

Each serving:
209 calories
9 calories from fat
1 g fat
0 g saturated fat
3 g protein
54 g carbohydrates

1. Rinse apples and cut into sixths. Scrub beets; discard tops if wilted or use them if not. Rinse and quarter pear. Peel lemon.

2. Push apples, beets, pear, lemon, and ginger through the juicer, and process until juiced. Stir well and pour juice into two glasses.

3. Serve immediately, garnished with apple wedges if desired.

Variation: To pulp this recipe in a blender or food processor fitted with a steel blade, core apple and pear, remove seeds from lemon, and cut all ingredients into pieces no larger than 1 inch.

Pulp Tidbits

Ginger is native to Asia and was well known to Europeans back in the Roman Era. It was highly valued and fifteen times more expensive than prized black peppercorns. It disappeared from Europe during the Middle Ages, but it was one of the crops Marco Polo brought back from his explorations; thus it was reestablished on that continent.

Strawberry and Beet

1 pt. strawberries

1 large beet

2 celery ribs

1 cup plain nonfat yogurt

¼ cup fruit-only strawberry jam

2 strawberries for garnish (optional)

Serves 2
Prep time: less than 10 minutes
Each serving: 253 calories 9 calories from fat 1 g fat 0 g saturated fat 9 g protein 54 g carbohydrates

1. Rinse strawberries. Scrub beets well, discard tops if wilted but rinse and use if not, and cut into 2-inch cubes. Rinse celery, and cut into 2-inch lengths.

2. Push strawberries, beet, and celery through the juicer, and process until juiced. Pour juice into a blender, and add yogurt and jam. Blend for 30 seconds, and pour juice into two glasses.

3. Serve immediately, garnished with strawberries if desired.

Variation: To pulp this recipe in a blender or food processor fitted with a steel blade, remove tops from strawberries and cut all ingredients into pieces no larger than 1 inch. If using a blender or food processor, add yogurt and jam with other ingredients.

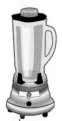

Wrong Spin! _____

Beets, along with carrots, can be toxic if eaten in too large a quantity. When making juices with these vegetables, do not double up on the quantities or eat other forms of these vegetables within a few hours.

Orange, Carrot, and Fennel

4 oranges

2 carrots

1 fennel bulb

¼ lime

2 orange slices for garnish (optional)

Serves 2
Prep time: less than 10 minutes
Each serving: 191 calories 9 calories from fat 1 g fat 0 g saturated fat 5 g protein 47 g carbohydrates

1. Peel and quarter oranges. Scrub carrots, discard tops, and cut into 2-inch lengths. Rinse fennel, trim stem end, and cut into 2-inch cubes. Peel lime.

2. Push oranges, carrots, fennel, and lime through the juicer, and process until juiced. Stir well and pour juice into two glasses.

3. Serve immediately, garnished with orange slices if desired.

Variation: To pulp this recipe in a blender or food processor fitted with a steel blade, remove seeds from oranges and lime and cut all ingredients into pieces no larger than 1 inch.

Juicy Jive

Fennel gives juices, and all raw dishes, a delightful anise flavor similar to a mild licorice. But if you're a person who doesn't care for licorice or any food in the anise family, you can always substitute celery in juice recipes.

Mixed Fruit and Tomato

4 ripe plum tomatoes

1 pt. strawberries

1 mango

¼ lemon

2 strawberries for garnish (optional)

Serves 2
Prep time: less than 10 minutes
Each serving: 171 calories 18 calories from fat 2 g fat 0 g saturated fat 4 g protein 42 g carbohydrates

1. Rinse and quarter tomatoes. Rinse strawberries. Peel mango, discard seed, and cut into 2-inch cubes. Peel lemon.

2. Push tomatoes, strawberries, mango, and lemon through the juicer, and process until juiced. Stir well and pour juice into two glasses.

3. Serve immediately, garnished with strawberries if desired.

Variation: To pulp this recipe in a blender or food processor fitted with a steel blade, core tomato, remove seeds from lemon, and cut all ingredients into pieces no larger than 1 inch.

Pulp Tidbits

It's hard to imagine today that three popular foods—tomatoes, potatoes, and eggplant—were all considered poisonous in the sixteenth century. The problem was that people were eating the leaves and stalks and not the fruit or tuber. And, indeed, the leaves of all three are toxic.

Carrot and Strawberry

4 carrots

2 celery ribs

1 pt. strawberries

1 cup strawberry nonfat yogurt

2 carrot sticks for garnish (optional)

Serves 2

Prep time:
less than 10 minutes

Each serving:
168 calories
9 calories from fat
1 g fat
0 g saturated fat
6 g protein
36 g carbohydrates

1. Scrub carrots, discard tops, and cut into 2-inch lengths. Rinse celery and cut into 2-inch lengths. Rinse strawberries.

2. Push carrots, celery, and strawberries through the juicer, and process until juiced. Pour juice into a blender and add yogurt. Blend for 30 seconds, and pour juice into two glasses.

3. Serve immediately, garnished with carrot sticks if desired.

Variation: To pulp this recipe in a blender or food processor fitted with a steel blade, remove tops from strawberries and cut all ingredients into pieces no larger than 1 inch. If using a blender or food processor, add yogurt with other ingredients.

Juicy Jive

Flavored yogurt is a great time-saver. But if you don't want to add refined sugar to your diet, you can achieve the same flavor by mixing 2 tablespoons of fruit-only jam into each 8-ounce container of plain yogurt.

Spiced Apple and Butternut Squash

4 apples

½ butternut squash

1 carrot

¼ tsp. ground cinnamon

⅛ tsp. ground nutmeg

2 apple wedges for garnish (optional)

Serves 2
Prep time: less than 10 minutes
Each serving: 265 calories 9 calories from fat 1 g fat 0 g saturated fat 3 g protein 69 g carbohydrates

1. Rinse apples and cut into sixths. Peel squash and cut into 2-inch cubes. Scrub carrot, discard top, and cut into 2-inch lengths.

2. Push apples, squash, and carrot through the juicer, and process until juiced. Pour juice into two glasses, and stir ⅛ tsp. cinnamon and ¹⁄₁₆ tsp. nutmeg into each glass.

3. Serve immediately, garnished with apple wedges if desired.

Variation: To pulp this recipe in a blender or food processor fitted with a steel blade, core apples and cut all ingredients into pieces no larger than 1 inch. If using a blender or food processor, add cinnamon and nutmeg with other ingredients.

Juicy Jive

Acorn and butternut squash are distinct species, and look nothing alike in the produce section. However, they have a flavor that's almost identical to one another, so use them interchangeably in any recipe.

Pineapple and Yam

¼ pineapple

2 apples

2 celery ribs

1 yams

2 pineapple spears for garnish (optional)

Serves 2
Prep time: less than 10 minutes
Each serving: 223 calories 9 calories from fat 1 g fat 0 g saturated fat 2 g protein 56 g carbohydrates

1. Cut pineapple off rind and into 2-inch cubes. Rinse apples and cut into sixths. Rinse celery and cut into 2-inch lengths. Scrub yam well, and cut into 2-inch cubes.

2. Push pineapple, apples, celery, and yam through the juicer, and process until juiced. Stir well and pour juice into two glasses.

3. Serve immediately, garnished with pineapple spears if desired.

Variation: To pulp this recipe in a blender or food processor fitted with a steel blade, core apples, peel yam, and cut all ingredients into pieces no larger than 1 inch.

Pulp Tidbits ────────────────────────────────

The use of the pineapple as a symbol of hospitality dates back to the time when the Spaniards first encountered it in the Caribbean. The Carib Indians would hang pineapple crowns outside their huts to show that visitors were welcome.

Mango and Orange Bell Pepper

3 orange bell peppers

2 celery ribs

1 mango

1 orange

¼ lime

2 orange bell pepper slices for garnish (optional)

Serves 2
Prep time: less than 10 minutes
Each serving: 144 calories 9 calories from fat 1 g fat 0 g saturated fat 3 g protein 36 g carbohydrates

1. Discard cap and seeds from pepper, and cut into 2-inch pieces. Rinse celery and cut into 2-inch lengths. Peel mango, discard seed, and cut into 2-inch cubes. Peel and quarter orange. Peel lime.

2. Push peppers, celery, mango, orange, and lime through the juicer, and process until juiced. Stir well and pour juice into two glasses.

3. Serve immediately, garnished with bell pepper slices if desired.

Variation: To pulp this recipe in a blender or food processor fitted with a steel blade, remove seeds from orange and lime and cut all ingredients into pieces no larger than 1 inch.

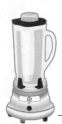

Wrong Spin! _____

This is one recipe you should follow closely. If you use green peppers or even red peppers instead of the orange peppers, the juice has a most unappealing color!

Part 3

Fruity and Fantastic

Picture Carmen Miranda, or Chiquita Banana for that matter, with a colorful headdress of fruit and a samba playing in the background. Fruits are nature's succulent gifts, and the recipes you'll find in this part glorify them.

Juices are almost synonymous with fruit, and juicing is a great way to enjoy and combine them. The recipes are divided by which type of fruit comprises the largest percentage of the juice, but you can always add other fruits to the mix and get delicious results.

Chapter **10**

Tree-Ripened Treats

In This Chapter

- ◆ Juices based on ever-popular apples
- ◆ Spectacular summertime juices with peaches and pears
- ◆ Great ways with grapes

This chapter features recipes that highlight fruits that come from deciduous trees and vines. So for Americans in the summer and fall, these crops will be local and lively.

While pears are better ripened off the tree so they don't turn mealy (a botanical fact that aids their transportation as well), all other fruits reach their peak of flavor when they're allowed to ripen attached to the tree on which they were grown.

Feel free to use the large range of recipes in this chapter as a springboard to your own concoctions. For example, if you have nectarines locally but not peaches, then feel free to experiment.

Blossoms to Bounty

A fruit tree is basically any tree that forms fruit in the ripened ovary of a flower containing at least one seed. But over the centuries we've come to use the term only for trees that produce fruit that humans eat. In the larger sense, nut trees, such as walnut and pecan, can also be considered fruit trees.

This fruit is produced in a form of botanical sex through a process called pollination. Pollination is the transfer of pollen, which is the male part of the flower, to the stigma, which is the female part of the flower. This transfer of pollen is needed for fruit to set and seeds to develop.

For this process, the honey bee is the trees' best friend. And this is why honey is classified by the pollen the bees have moved around—ranging from common clover to exotic orange blossom or lavender.

Vintage Vines

While grapes grow on woody vines rather than trees, their fruit falls into the same category as that of deciduous trees. Literally thousands of varieties of grapes are grown, divided by color as well as by purpose.

In general, the wine varietals like cabernet or chardonnay are not pleasant to eat off the vine because of the same high acid content that creates complexity in wine. Conversely, table grapes with low acidity would make very bland wine. While concord grapes are the ones most often used in grape juice, they're hard to find in supermarkets.

Gingered Apple and Pear

3 apples

3 ripe pears

2 TB. sliced fresh ginger

2 tsp. hoisin sauce

2 apple slices for garnish (optional)

Serves 2

Prep time:
less than 10 minutes

Each serving:
273 calories
9 calories from fat
1 g fat
0 g saturated fat
2 g protein
72 g carbohydrates

1. Rinse apples and cut into sixths. Rinse and quarter pears.

2. Push apples, pears, and ginger through the juicer, and process until juiced. Pour juice into two glasses. Stir 1 teaspoon of *hoisin sauce* into each glass.

3. Serve immediately, garnished with apple slices if desired.

Variation: To pulp this recipe in a blender or food processor fitted with a steel blade, core apples and pears, peel ginger, and cut all ingredients into pieces no larger than 1 inch.

Liquid Lingo ⸺

Hoisin sauce is a soybean-based thick sauce with a sweet and spicy flavor. Used in many Chinese dishes, it also includes garlic, chili peppers, and some form of sugar or honey.

Grape, Orange, and Carrot

3 cups green or red seedless grapes

1 orange

1 apple

¼ lime

2 orange slices for garnish (optional)

Serves 2

Prep time:
less than 10 minutes

Each serving:
239 calories
9 calories from fat
1 g fat
0 g saturated fat
3 g protein
63 g carbohydrates

1. Rinse grapes. Peel and quarter orange. Rinse apple and cut into sixths. Peel lime.

2. Push grapes, orange, apple, and lime through the juicer, and process until juiced. Stir well and pour juice into two glasses.

3. Serve immediately, garnished with orange slices if desired.

Variation: To pulp this recipe in a blender or food processor fitted with a steel blade, core apple, remove seeds from lime, and cut all ingredients into pieces no larger than 1 inch.

Juicy Jive

We use small amounts of tart citrus juices like lemon and lime in many recipes to boost the flavor of the other ingredients. You won't taste the lime as much as you'll have a sensation of a vivid taste.

Peach and Pear

3 peaches

3 pears

1 apple

¼ fennel bulb

2 peach slices for garnish (optional)

Serves 2
Prep time: less than 10 minutes
Each serving: 249 calories 9 calories from fat 1 g fat 0 g saturated fat 3 g protein 65 g carbohydrates

1. Rinse peaches, discard stones, and cut into quarters. Rinse pears and cut into quarters. Rinse apple and cut into sixths. Rinse fennel, trim stem end, and cut into 2-inch cubes.

2. Push peaches, pears, apple, and fennel through the juicer, and process until juiced. Stir well and pour juice into two glasses.

3. Serve immediately, garnished with peach slices if desired.

Variation: To pulp this recipe in a blender or food processor fitted with a steel blade, core pears and apple and cut all ingredients into pieces no larger than 1 inch.

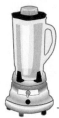

Wrong Spin!

While the seeds of some fruits, such as grapes or oranges, might be unpleasant to eat, peach pits can be toxic. Always be sure to discard the stone as well as the seed before juicing peaches.

Peach and Pomegranate

3 peaches

1 pomegranate

1 apple

1 TB. honey

½ cup crushed ice

2 peach slices for garnish (optional)

Serves 2

Prep time:
less than 10 minutes

Each serving:
180 calories
9 calories from fat
1 g fat
0 g saturated fat
2 g protein
46 g carbohydrates

1. Rinse peaches, discard stones, and cut into quarters. Break pomegranate apart, pull out red pulp, and discard rind. Rinse apple and cut into sixths.

2. Push peaches, pomegranate, and apple through the juicer, and process until juiced. Pour juice into a blender and add honey and ice. Blend for 30 seconds. Stir well and pour juice into two glasses.

3. Serve immediately, garnished with peach slices if desired.

Variation: To pulp this recipe in a blender or food processor fitted with a steel blade, cut all ingredients into pieces no larger than 1 inch. If using a blender or food processor, add honey and ice along with other ingredients, and strain mixture to remove pomegranate seeds.

Pulp Tidbits

The pomegranate is a fruit specifically mentioned in the Bible. One of the Songs of Solomon contains the line "Thou art fair, my love. Thy temples are like a piece of pomegranate within thy locks." It's also mentioned that King Solomon kept a grove of pomegranate trees.

Plum and Pear

6 plums

2 pears

12 prunes

Pinch of cinnamon

2 plum slices for garnish (optional)

Serves 2
Prep time: less than 10 minutes
Each serving: 311 calories 9 calories from fat 1 g fat 0 g saturated fat 3 g protein 81 g carbohydrates

1. Rinse plums, discard stones, and cut in half. Rinse and quarter pears.

2. Push plums and pears through the juicer, and process until juiced. Pour juice into a blender and add prunes and *pinch* of cinnamon. Blend for 30 seconds, and pour juice into two glasses.

3. Serve immediately, garnished with plum slices if desired.

Variation: To pulp this recipe in a blender or food processor fitted with a steel blade, core pears and cut all ingredients into pieces no larger than 1 inch. If using a blender or food processor, add prunes and cinnamon along with other ingredients.

Liquid Lingo

Pinch is a measuring term that refers to the amount of a dry ingredient that can be held between the tips of the thumb and forefinger. It's equivalent to approximately 1/16 teaspoon.

Grape, Pear, and Lychee

3 cups green seedless grapes

2 pears

1 apple

36 lychees

¼ tsp. ground cinnamon

2 pear slices for garnish (optional)

Serves 2
Prep time: less than 10 minutes
Each serving: 419 calories 9 calories from fat 1 g fat 0 g saturated fat 4 g protein 109 carbohydrates

1. Rinse grapes. Rinse pears and cut into quarters. Rinse apple and cut into sixths. Peel *lychees* apart, and discard seeds.

2. Push grapes, pears, apple, and lychees through the juicer, and process until juiced. Pour juice into two glasses, and stir ⅛ teaspoon cinnamon into each.

3. Serve immediately, garnished with pear slices if desired.

Variation: To pulp this recipe in a blender or food processor fitted with a steel blade, core pears and apple and cut all ingredients into pieces no larger than 1 inch.

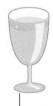

Liquid Lingo

Lychees, sometimes called lychee nuts, are an ancient Chinese fruit. Round and about 1 inch in diameter, a rough, bright red shell protects the juicy sweet flesh. They're only found fresh in the late spring, but they can be used canned as well.

Grape, Kiwi, and Orange

1½ cups green or red seedless grapes

6 kiwis

2 oranges

2 celery ribs

2 orange slices for garnish (optional)

Serves 2
Prep time: less than 10 minutes
Each serving: 293 calories 9 calories from fat 1 g fat 0 g saturated fat 5 g protein 73 g carbohydrates

1. Rinse grapes and kiwis. Peel and quarter oranges. Rinse celery and cut into 2-inch lengths.

2. Push grapes, kiwis, oranges, and celery through the juicer, and process until juiced. Stir well and pour juice into two glasses.

3. Serve immediately, garnished with orange slices if desired.

Variation: To pulp this recipe in a blender or food processor fitted with a steel blade, peel kiwis, remove seeds from oranges, and cut all ingredients into pieces no larger than 1 inch.

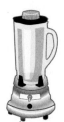

Wrong Spin!

If you're using a juicer for this or any recipe that includes grapes, it doesn't matter if they're seedless or have seeds. But if you're going to pulp a recipe with grapes, always make sure the grapes are seedless, and Thompson grapes are the most common variety. The pesky seeds will not purée, and to manually discard them will take a lot of time.

Peach, Apricot, and Raspberry

3 peaches

6 apricots

1 (½ pt.) container raspberries

½ cup apricot nectar

2 peach slices for garnish (optional)

Serves 2

Prep time:
less than 10 minutes

Each serving:
241 calories
18 calories from fat
2 g fat
0 g saturated fat
5 g protein
57 g carbohydrates

1. Rinse peaches, discard stones, and cut into quarters. Rinse and halve apricots, discarding stones. Rinse raspberries.

2. Push peaches, apricots, and raspberries through the juicer, and process until juiced. Pour juice into two glasses, and stir ¼ cup apricot nectar into each.

3. Serve immediately, garnished with peach slices if desired.

Variation: To pulp this recipe in a blender or food processor fitted with a steel blade, cut all ingredients into pieces no larger than 1 inch, and add, apricot nectar along with the other ingredients.

Juicy Jive

One of the great advantages of a juicer is that all the tiny seeds in berries, which can aggravate conditions such as diverticulitis, are strained out in the process. When using a food processor or blender, it's best to strain any berry drinks.

Tangerine, Grape, and Pineapple

4 tangerines

1½ cups red seedless grapes

¼ pineapple

¼ lime

2 pineapple spears for garnish (optional)

Serves 2
Prep time:
less than 10 minutes
Each serving:
243 calories
9 calories from fat
1 g fat
0 g saturated fat
3 g protein
63 g carbohydrates

1. Peel tangerines and break into quarters. Rinse grapes. Cut rind off pineapple and cut into 2-inch cubes. Peel lime.

2. Push tangerines, grapes, pineapple, and lime through the juicer, and process until juiced. Stir well and pour juice into two glasses.

3. Serve immediately, garnished with pineapple spears if desired.

Variation: To pulp this recipe in a blender or food processor fitted with a steel blade, remove seeds from lime and cut all ingredients into pieces no larger than 1 inch.

Pulp Tidbits

Named for Tangier, Morocco, tangerines are the most common member of the mandarin orange family found in the United States, which also includes tiny clementines. What distinguishes these species of fruit is that the skins are loose and slip off easily.

Gingered Apricot, Peach, and Orange

10 ripe apricots

2 peaches

1 orange

2 TB. sliced fresh ginger

½ cup dried apricots

2 apricot wedges for garnish (optional)

Serves 2
Prep time:
less than 10 minutes
Each serving:
203 calories
9 calories from fat
1 g fat
0 g saturated fat
4 g protein
51 g carbohydrates

1. Rinse apricots, cut in half, discarding stones. Rinse peaches, discard stones, and cut into quarters. Peel and quarter orange.

2. Push apricots, peaches, orange, and ginger through the juicer, and process until juiced. Pour juice into a blender and add apricots. Blend for 30 seconds, and pour juice into two glasses.

3. Serve immediately, garnished with apricot wedges if desired.

Variation: To pulp this recipe in a blender or food processor fitted with a steel blade, remove seeds from oranges, peel ginger, and cut all ingredients into pieces no larger than 1 inch. If using a blender or food processor, add apricots along with other ingredients.

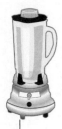

Wrong Spin!

Make sure your dried apricots or any dried fruit is unsulphured, which means it has not been sprayed with sulphur dioxide, a gas used for fumigation that destroys the fruit's B vitamins. Most health food stores are good sources for naturally dried fruits, but even fruit that is organic might be sprayed.

Chapter

11

It's the Berries!

In This Chapter

- ◆ Bright juices with vividly colored strawberries
- ◆ Intensely flavored juices made with blackberries
- ◆ Juices featuring all-American cranberries and blueberries

Come summer, nothing is better than fresh berries from a farm stand, and you'll find recipes for juices glorifying their vivid colors and luscious flavors in this chapter. While modern transportation has made it possible to enjoy these fruits during any month of the year, berries are the most affordable and at their peak of ripeness during warm weather.

Berries are good sources of vitamins and are on the list of foods high in disease-fighting antioxidants. Also, in their juiced form, they don't contain any pesky little seeds, which, of course, is another benefit.

Confusing Clan

In a trivia contest if you were shown a strawberry and a tomato and asked which was the berry, you—like all of us—would probably opt for the wrong answer. In botany berries are simple fleshy fruits, so the tomato, as well as the eggplant and avocado, qualifies. But in common usage a berry is a small, sweet fruit with many seeds.

While the blueberry and the cranberry are actual berries, the strawberry is termed a false berry because we eat the material that surrounds the seeds. Both raspberries and blackberries are actually clusters of tiny fruits held together by common walls. That's why they are hollow in the center.

Garnishing Greatness

You've probably noticed that all the garnishes suggested for the juice drinks in this book are an ingredient comprising the mix. And that's true for the recipes in this chapter, too, but tiny fruits like raspberries are just too little to stay perched on a glass.

For a strawberry garnish, rinse the strawberry and cut it from the tip halfway up to the green top. Then you can secure it to the side of the glass.

For smaller berries, the only way they won't get lost in the juice is if they're placed on skewers. Any long toothpick will do, and those with the frilled cellophane tips used to secure sandwiches are the best.

Spiced Cranberry and Apple

3 cups cranberries

4 apples

3 TB. honey

½ tsp. ground cinnamon

¼ tsp. ground nutmeg

2 apple slices for garnish (optional)

Serves 2
Prep time:
less than 10 minutes
Each serving:
323 calories
9 calories from fat
1 g fat
0 g saturated fat
1 g protein
86 g carbohydrates

1. Rinse cranberries. Rinse apples and cut into sixths.

2. Push cranberries and apples through the juicer, and process until juiced. Pour juice into two glasses, add 1½ tablespoons honey, ¼ teaspoon cinnamon, and ⅛ teaspoon nutmeg to each glass, and stir well.

3. Serve immediately, garnished with apple slices if desired.

Variation: To pulp this recipe in a blender or food processor fitted with a steel blade, core apples and cut all ingredients into pieces no larger than 1 inch. If using a blender or food processor, add honey, cinnamon, and nutmeg along with other ingredients.

Pulp Tidbits

Cranberries are native to the Cape Cod area, and it's possible the Pilgrims were brought a condiment in some form at the first Thanksgiving dinner in 1621. But our word cranberry is not English; it's a corruption from the Dutch kranbeere, or craneberry, because the stamen resembled a beak.

Gingered Strawberry and Rhubarb

1 quart strawberries

3 (8-inch) rhubarb stalks

1 orange

3 TB. sliced ginger

3 TB. honey

2 strawberries for garnish (optional)

Serves 2
Prep time:
less than 10 minutes
Each serving:
246 calories
9 calories from fat
1 g fat
0 g saturated fat
4 g protein
62 g carbohydrates

1. Rinse strawberries. Rinse rhubarb and cut into 2-inch lengths. Peel and quarter orange.

2. Push strawberries, rhubarb, orange, and ginger through the juicer, and process until juiced. Pour juice into two glasses, and stir 1½ tablespoons honey into each glass.

3. Serve immediately, garnished with strawberries if desired.

Variation: To pulp this recipe in a blender or food processor fitted with a steel blade, remove green tops from strawberries, peel ginger, and cut all ingredients into pieces no larger than 1 inch. If using a blender or food processor, add honey along with other ingredients.

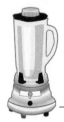

Wrong Spin!

If someone gives you home-grown rhubarb, discard all traces of the leaves before juicing or cooking it. Even though the fluffy leaves resemble those of kale, they are very toxic.

Strawberry, Grape, and Cucumber

1 pint strawberries

1½ cups seedless red grapes

2 apples

½ cucumber

2 strawberries for garnish (optional)

Serves 2
Prep time: less than 10 minutes
Each serving: 216 calories 9 calories from fat 1 g fat 0 g saturated fat 3 g protein 55 g carbohydrates

1. Rinse strawberries and grapes. Rinse apples and cut into sixths. Rinse cucumber and cut into 2-inch lengths.

2. Push strawberries, grapes, apples, and cucumber through the juicer, and process until juiced. Stir well and pour juice into two glasses.

3. Serve immediately, garnished with strawberries if desired.

Variation: To pulp this recipe in a blender or food processor fitted with a steel blade, remove tops from strawberries, core apple, and cut all ingredients into pieces no larger than 1 inch.

Juicy Jive

In a juice such as this one, the vibrant flavor of the fruits will eclipse the subtle flavor of the cucumber, but that's its purpose in the recipe. It adds nutrients while letting the fruits take the starring role.

Strawberry, Pineapple, and Passion Fruit

1 pint strawberries

¼ pineapple

4 passion fruit

¼ lime

2 pineapple spears for garnish (optional)

Serves 2
Prep time: less than 10 minutes
Each serving: 152 calories 9 calories from fat 1 g fat 0 g saturated fat 3 g protein 38 g carbohydrates

1. Rinse strawberries. Cut rind off pineapple, and cut fruit into 2-inch cubes. Rinse and halve passion fruit. Peel lime.

2. Push strawberries, pineapple, passion fruit, and lime through the juicer, and process until juiced. Stir well and pour juice into two glasses.

3. Serve immediately, garnished with pineapple spears if desired.

Variation: To pulp this recipe in a blender or food processor fitted with a steel blade, remove tops from strawberries, peel passion fruit, remove seeds from lime, and cut all ingredients into pieces no larger than 1 inch.

Pulp Tidbits

Passion fruit, native to Brazil, did not get its name because it was rumored to have aphrodisiac qualities. The passion in question is Christ's crucifixion, because the flower on the tree resembles the Crown of Thorns.

Spiced Blueberry and Banana

1½ cups blueberries

2 pears

2 bananas

1 cup plain soy milk

2 pear wedges for garnish (optional)

Serves 2
Prep time: less than 10 minutes
Each serving: 319 calories 27 calories from fat 3 g fat 0 g saturated fat 6 g protein 74 g carbohydrates

1. Rinse blueberries. Rinse pears and cut into quarters. Peel and slice bananas.

2. Push blueberries and pears through the juicer, and process until juiced. Pour juice into a blender and add bananas and *soy milk*. Blend for 30 seconds, and pour juice into two glasses.

3. Serve immediately, garnished with pear wedges if desired.

Variation: To pulp this recipe in a blender or food processor fitted with a steel blade, core pears and cut all ingredients into pieces no larger than 1 inch. If using a blender or food processor, add bananas and soy milk along with other ingredients.

Liquid Lingo

Soy milk is an iron-rich liquid made by pressing soybeans that are ground and cooked. It's higher in protein than cow's milk, and it's nondairy so people who have milk allergies can digest it. It's not as high in calcium as cow's milk, but many brands are fortified with calcium.

Blueberry, Strawberry, and Apple

1 qt. blueberries

1 pt. strawberries

2 apples

¼ lemon

2 strawberries for garnish (optional)

Serves 2
Prep time: less than 10 minutes
Each serving: 288 calories 18 calories from fat 2 g fat 0 g saturated fat 4 g protein 73 g carbohydrates

1. Rinse blueberries and strawberries. Rinse apples and cut into sixths. Peel lemon.

2. Push strawberries, blueberries, apples, and lemon through the juicer, and process until juiced. Stir well and pour juice into two glasses.

3. Serve immediately, garnished with strawberries if desired.

Variation: To pulp this recipe in a blender or food processor fitted with a steel blade, core apples, remove lemon seeds, and cut all ingredients into pieces no larger than 1 inch.

Pulp Tidbits

There are actually a few types of blueberries, which are a crop native to North America. The famed wild blueberries of Maine are tiny and come from low bushes. Most of the crop is still hand-picked using a rake invented in 1822. The majority of today's blueberries are much larger high-bush berries, with New Jersey, Michigan, and Washington leading in cultivation.

Raspberry, Cranberry, and Grape

1½ pts. raspberries

2 cups seedless red grapes

1 cup cranberries

2 TB. superfine granulated sugar

2 skewers of raspberries for garnish (optional)

Serves 2
Prep time:
less than 10 minutes
Each serving:
283 calories
18 calories from fat
2 g fat
0 g saturated fat
4 g protein
71 g carbohydrates

1. Rinse raspberries, grapes, and cranberries.

2. Push raspberries, grapes, and cranberries through the juicer, and process until juiced. Pour juice into two glasses, and stir 1 tablespoon sugar into each.

3. Serve immediately, garnished with skewers of raspberries if desired.

Variation: To pulp this recipe in a blender or food processor fitted with a steel blade, add sugar along with other ingredients.

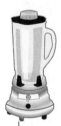

Wrong Spin!

Don't confuse superfine sugar with confectioners' sugar. Superfine is finely granulated to dissolve almost instantly, which is why it's a good addition to juices. Confectioners' sugar is also finely granulated but has cornstarch added to prevent it from clumping.

Mixed Berry and Pear

1 pt. strawberries

½ pt. raspberries

½ pt. blackberries

3 pears

2 mixed-berry skewers for garnish
(optional)

Serves 2
Prep time:
less than 10 minutes
Each serving:
257 calories
14 calories from fat
1.5 g fat
0 g saturated fat
4 g protein
65 g carbohydrates

1. Rinse strawberries, raspberries, and blackberries. Rinse and quarter pears.

2. Push strawberries, raspberries, blackberries, and pears through the juicer, and process until juiced. Stir well and pour juice into two glasses.

3. Serve immediately, garnished with mixed-berry skewers if desired.

Variation: To pulp this recipe in a blender or food processor fitted with a steel blade, remove tops from strawberries, core pears, and cut all ingredients into pieces no larger than 1 inch.

Juicy Jive

You can use any combination of berries for this recipe, as long as the quantity remains the same. The pear produces a creamy quality in contrast to the vivid flavor of the berries, but choose whatever berries look best in the market.

Blackberry, Grape, and Banana

1½ pts. blackberries

2 cups red seedless grapes

2 bananas

2 skewers of blackberries for garnish (optional)

Serves 2

Prep time:
less than 10 minutes

Each serving:
312 calories
18 calories from fat
2 g fat
0 g saturated fat
6 g protein
77.5 g carbohydrates

1. Rinse blackberries and grapes. Peel and slice bananas.

2. Push blackberries and grapes through the juicer, and process until juiced. Pour juice into a blender, and add bananas. Blend for 30 seconds, and pour juice into two glasses.

3. Serve immediately, garnished with skewers of blackberries if desired.

Variation: To pulp this recipe in a blender or food processor fitted with a steel blade, add bananas along with other ingredients.

Juicy Jive

Blackberries and raspberries are the most delicate berries. Not only do they bruise and break easily, but they also mold rapidly once they've been bruised. When selecting them at the market, turn the package over. If there's a lot of color, the berries have been broken.

Sparkling Blackberry, Mango, and Lemon

1½ pts. blackberries

2 mangoes

¼ lemon

¾ cup sparkling mineral water

2 mango spears for garnish (optional)

Serves 2
Prep time: less than 10 minutes
Each serving: 238 calories 18 calories from fat 2 g fat 0 g saturated fat 4 g protein 59 g carbohydrates

1. Rinse blackberries. Peel mangoes, discard stones, and cut fruit into 2-inch pieces. Peel lemon.

2. Push blackberries, mangoes, and lemon through the juicer, and process until juiced. Pour juice into two glasses, and stir ⅜ cup sparkling water into each.

3. Serve immediately, garnished with mango spears if desired.

Variation: To pulp this recipe in a blender or food processor fitted with a steel blade, remove seeds from lemon and cut all ingredients into pieces no larger than 1 inch.

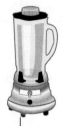

Wrong Spin!

Mangoes are actually part of the same family as poison ivy; both contain a chemical substance known as urushiol. When handling a mango, if you find your hands becoming irritated, wear rubber gloves. Some people are more sensitive to the urushiol than others. However, the chemical is only in the skin and not in the fruit, so everyone can eat mangoes.

Chapter 12

Make Mine Melon

In This Chapter

- ◆ Juices for cantaloupe cravings
- ◆ Drinks if you're wild for watermelon
- ◆ Making it happen with honeydew

Melons are always thirst-quenching because they're more than 90 percent water. So it's not surprising that they are great as the base fruit for juices, and recipes using melons are what you'll find in this chapter.

Melons are mild in flavor, so they're used as a larger proportion of the fruit than the combinations used in other chapters. But it's amazing how delicious they are when combined with other fruits.

When juicing, there's no need to discard the melon seeds, which both saves time and boosts flavor. A melon's sweetest flesh is the part that surrounds the seeds.

Nature's Lucky Trick

Melons grow on long vines and have been cultivated for more than 4,000 years, although the now-popular honeydew is a recent hybrid. The fact that we have them is a trick of nature called a false berry.

The actual fruit of the vine is the pesky seeds we discard when we eat the melon. The luscious flesh is the accessory to the seeds.

Names for melons change from continent to continent. What we call a cantaloupe is dubbed a musk melon in most English-speaking countries, and our honeydew is a White Antibes in Europe.

Cantaloupe, Blueberry, and Cherry

½ cantaloupe

2 cups blueberries

1½ cups cherries

½ banana

1 TB. blueberry jam

2 cantaloupe slices for garnish (optional)

Serves 2
Prep time: less than 10 minutes
Each serving: 272 calories 9 calories from fat 1 g fat 0 g saturated fat 4 g protein 68 g carbohydrates

1. Peel cantaloupe and cut into 2-inch cubes. Rinse blueberries. Rinse and pit cherries.

2. Push cantaloupe, blueberries, and cherries through the juicer, and process until juiced. Pour juice into a blender, and add banana and jam. Blend for 30 seconds. Stir well, and pour juice into two glasses.

3. Serve immediately, garnished with cantaloupe slices if desired.

Variation: To pulp this recipe in a blender or food processor fitted with a steel blade, discard cantaloupe seeds, and cut all ingredients into pieces no larger than 1 inch. If using a blender or food processor, add banana and jam along with other ingredients.

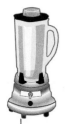

Wrong Spin!

Cantaloupes have been known to carry salmonella bacteria on their rinds, and this bacteria can be transferred to the flesh when the melon is cut. Always wash a cantaloupe with soap and water and rinse it well before cutting it open.

Cantaloupe, Apricot, and Carrot

$\frac{1}{2}$ cantaloupe

6 fresh apricots

2 carrots

$\frac{1}{2}$ cup dried apricots

2 slices cantaloupe for garnish (optional)

Serves 2
Prep time: less than 10 minutes
Each serving: 193 calories 9 calories from fat 1 g fat 0 g saturated fat 4 g protein 47 g carbohydrates

1. Peel cantaloupe and cut into 2-inch cubes. Rinse and halve apricots, and discard stones. Scrub carrots, discard tops, and cut into 2-inch lengths.

2. Push cantaloupe, apricots, and carrots through the juicer, and process until juiced. Pour juice into a blender and add dried apricots. Blend for 30 seconds, and pour juice into two glasses.

3. Serve immediately, garnished with cantaloupe slices if desired.

Variation: To pulp this recipe in a blender or food processor fitted with a steel blade, discard cantaloupe seeds, and cut all ingredients into pieces no larger than 1 inch. If using a blender or food processor, add dried apricots along with other ingredients.

Pulp Tidbits

The modern American cantaloupe is a new kid. The W. Atlee Burpee Company developed and introduced it in 1881 under the name "Netted Gem" because the rind resembled a type of netting.

Spiced Cantaloupe and Pear

¹/₂ cantaloupe

3 pears

¹/₂ cup silken tofu

Pinch of ground cinnamon

Pinch of ground allspice

2 cinnamon sticks for garnish (optional)

Serves 2
Prep time: less than 10 minutes
Each serving: 216 calories 9 calories from fat 1 g fat 0 g saturated fat 3 g protein 54 g carbohydrates

1. Peel cantaloupe and cut into 2-inch cubes. Rinse and quarter pears.

2. Push cantaloupe and pears through the juicer, and process until juiced. Pour juice into a blender, and add tofu, cinnamon, and allspice. Blend for 30 seconds. Pour juice into two glasses.

3. Serve immediately, garnished with cinnamon sticks if desired.

Variation: To pulp this recipe in a blender or food processor fitted with a steel blade, discard cantaloupe seeds, core pears, and cut all ingredients into pieces no larger than 1 inch. If using a blender or food processor, add tofu, cinnamon, and allspice along with other ingredients.

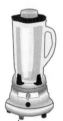

Wrong Spin!

While any of the species of pear listed in Chapter 2 will work for this or any other recipe for pears, be careful not to purchase Asian pears at the supermarket. Their flesh is crunchy like that of an apple without the rich sweetness of European pears.

Cantaloupe, Peach, and Yam

½ cantaloupe

3 peaches

2 yams

¼ tsp. ground cinnamon

2 peach slices for garnish (optional)

Serves 2

Prep time:
less than 10 minutes

Each serving:
261 calories
9 calories from fat
1 g fat
0 g saturated fat
5 g protein
62 g carbohydrates

1. Peel cantaloupe and cut into 2-inch cubes. Rinse peaches, discard stones, and cut into quarters. Scrub yams and cut into 2-inch cubes.

2. Push cantaloupe, peaches, and yams through the juicer, and process until juiced. Pour juice into two glasses, and stir ⅛ teaspoon cinnamon into each.

3. Serve immediately, garnished with peach slices if desired.

Variation: To pulp this recipe in a blender or food processor fitted with a steel blade, discard cantaloupe seeds, peel yams, and cut all ingredients into pieces no larger than 1 inch.

Juicy Jive

There is endless confusion between yams and sweet potatoes, and while you can cook the two interchangeably, they are from two different botanical species. Yams have a higher moisture content and are a bit sweeter than sweet potatoes. So if you're juicing a sweet potato rather than a yam, you might want to add a bit of molasses or brown sugar to the juice.

Watermelon and Berry Juice

1 pt. strawberries

½ pt. raspberries

½ cup cranberries

6 cups cubed watermelon without rind

2 watermelon spears for garnish (optional)

Serves 2
Prep time: less than 10 minutes
Each serving: 271 calories 18 calories from fat 2 g fat 0 g saturated fat 5 g protein 67 g carbohydrates

1. Rinse strawberries, raspberries, and cranberries. Push strawberries, raspberries, cranberries, and watermelon through the juicer, and process until juiced. Stir well, and pour juice into two glasses.

2. Serve immediately, garnished with watermelon spears if desired.

Variation: To pulp this recipe in a blender or food processor fitted with a steel blade, cut off strawberry tops, remove seeds from watermelon (if necessary), and cut all ingredients into pieces no larger than 1 inch.

Juicy Jive

If pulping rather than juicing this recipe, make sure that the watermelon is seedless before you buy it. If you find you have one with seeds, the best recourse is to briefly pulse the flesh in a food processor fitted with a steel blade, and the seeds will become easier to remove with a slotted spoon.

Watermelon, Peach, and Banana

3 peaches

2 bananas

6 cups cubed watermelon without rind

½ cup dried peaches

¼ tsp. ground cinnamon

2 watermelon spears for garnish (optional)

Serves 2
Prep time: less than 10 minutes
Each serving: 438 calories 18 calories from fat 2 g fat 0 g saturated fat 8 g protein 111 g carbohydrates

1. Rinse peaches, discard stones, and cut into quarters. Peel and slice bananas.

2. Push peaches and watermelon through the juicer, and process until juiced. Pour juice into a blender and add bananas, dried peaches, and cinnamon. Blend for 30 seconds, and pour juice into two glasses.

3. Serve immediately, garnished with watermelon spears if desired.

Variation: To pulp this recipe in a blender or food processor fitted with a steel blade, remove seeds from watermelon (if necessary) and cut all ingredients into pieces no larger than 1 inch. Add dried bananas, peaches, and cinnamon along with other ingredients.

Pulp Tidbits

While watermelons are African by birth, they play a large role in Mexican folklore, especially the Dia de los Muertos (Day of the Dead) celebrated on Halloween. Both in art and on ceramics watermelon is shown being eaten by the dead.

Watermelon, Raspberry, and Lemon

1 pint raspberries

1 apple

½ lemon

6 cups cubed watermelon without rind

2 watermelon spears for garnish (optional)

Serves 2
Prep time:
less than 10 minutes
Each serving:
284 calories
18 calories from fat
2 g fat
0 g saturated fat
5 g protein
71 g carbohydrates

1. Rinse raspberries. Rinse apple and cut into sixths. Peel lemon.

2. Push raspberries, apple, lemon, and watermelon through the juicer, and process until juiced. Stir well, and pour juice into two glasses.

3. Serve immediately, garnished with watermelon spears if desired.

Variation: To pulp this recipe in a blender or food processor fitted with a steel blade, core apple, remove lemon seeds, remove seeds from watermelon (if necessary), and cut all ingredients into pieces no larger than 1 inch.

Juicy Jive

When you're playing around with juicing different combinations, think about visual appeal. This juice, for example, is a blushing pink because the apple and lemon don't add color to the other fruit.

Honeydew, Kiwi, and Zucchini

¼ honeydew melon

4 kiwi fruit

1 cup green grapes

2 medium zucchini

2 celery ribs

2 honeydew slices for garnish (optional)

Serves 2
Prep time: less than 10 minutes
Each serving: 275 calories 18 calories from fat 2 g fat 0 g saturated fat 6 g protein 68 g carbohydrates

1. Peel honeydew melon and cut into 2-inch cubes. Rinse kiwis and grapes. Rinse zucchini and celery and cut into 2-inch lengths.

2. Push honeydew, kiwi, grapes, zucchini, and celery through the juicer, and process until juiced. Stir well and pour juice into two glasses.

3. Serve immediately, garnished with honeydew slices if desired.

Variation: To pulp this recipe in a blender or food processor fitted with a steel blade, discard honeydew seeds, peel kiwis, and cut all ingredients into pieces no larger than 1 inch.

Pulp Tidbits

The kiwi fruit is a case study in successful marketing. Their official name is Chinese gooseberries. They've been around for centuries and grown proudly in New Zealand. In the mid-1970s they were dubbed kiwi fruit, in honor of the flightless New Zealand bird, and suddenly their popularity skyrocketed in the United States.

Honeydew, Mango, and Citrus

¼ honeydew melon

2 mangoes

1 orange

¼ lemon

¼ lime

2 lemon or lime slice for garnish (optional)

Serves 2
Prep time:
less than 10 minutes
Each serving:
216 calories
9 calories from fat
1 g fat
0 g saturated fat
2.5 g protein
57 g carbohydrates

1. Peel honeydew and cut into 2-inch cubes. Peel mangoes, discard seed, and dice. Peel orange, lemon, and lime.

2. Push honeydew, mangoes, orange, lemon, and lime through the juicer, and process until juiced. Stir well and pour juice into two glasses.

3. Serve immediately, garnished with lemon or lime slices if desired.

Variation: To pulp this recipe in a blender or food processor fitted with a steel blade, discard honeydew seeds, remove seeds from orange, lemon, and lime, and cut all ingredients into pieces no larger than 1 inch.

Juicy Jive

If you're having problems peeling a mango, try peeling it from the other direction. Mangoes have an easy and hard way to peel, and it can vary from fruit to fruit.

Honeydew, Grape, and Cucumber

¼ honeydew melon

2 cups green grapes

1 cucumber

¼ lime

2 honeydew slices for garnish (optional)

Serves 2
Prep time:
less than 10 minutes
Each serving:
225 calories
9 calories from fat
1 g fat
0 g saturated fat
3.5 g protein
58 g carbohydrates

1. Peel honeydew and cut into 2-inch cubes. Rinse grapes. Rinse cucumber and cut into 2-inch lengths. Peel lime.

2. Push honeydew, grapes, cucumber, and lime through the juicer, and process until juiced. Stir well and pour juice into two glasses.

3. Serve immediately, garnished with honeydew slices if desired.

Variation: To pulp this recipe in a blender or food processor fitted with a steel blade, discard honeydew seeds, remove seeds from lime, and cut all ingredients into pieces no larger than 1 inch.

Juicy Jive

Selecting melons is never easy because they have such a hard rind. A general rule is to look at the stem end. It should smell sweet and be flat rather than indented. An indentation is a sign that the melon was pulled off the vine before it was ripe, at which time it comes off easily.

Minted Honeydew Citrus

¼ honeydew melon

1 grapefruit

2 celery ribs

¼ lemon

1 mint sprig

2 mint sprigs for garnish (optional)

Serves 2
Prep time: less than 10 minutes
Each serving: 106 calories 0 calories from fat 0 g fat 0 g saturated fat 2 g protein 27 g carbohydrates

1. Peel honeydew and cut into 2-inch cubes. Peel grapefruit and cut into sixths. Rinse celery and cut into 2-inch lengths. Peel lemon. Rinse mint sprig.

2. Push honeydew, oranges, celery, lemon, and *mint* through the juicer, and process until juiced. Stir well and pour juice into two glasses.

3. Serve immediately, garnished with mint sprigs if desired.

Variation: To pulp this recipe in a blender or food processor fitted with a steel blade, discard seeds from melon, remove seeds from grapefruit, and cut all ingredients into pieces no larger than 1 inch.

Liquid Lingo

Mint has more than 30 species, but peppermint and spearmint are the two most common. Peppermint, with bright green leaves and a peppery flavor, is the more pungent of the two. Spearmint's leaves are gray-green and much milder in both flavor and aroma.

Chapter 13

Tropical Treats

In This Chapter

- ◆ Sensational citrus juices
- ◆ Pineapple and papaya with panache
- ◆ Marvelous ways to enjoy mango

Drinking a tropical juice makes me feel as if I'm on vacation, with the heady aroma as a prelude to the sweet flavors. And by making some of these juice recipes, this vacation can take place at a moment's notice.

For most Americans, the arrival of tropical fruits other than Florida-grown citrus has been a relatively new development. Such fruits as papaya and mango were virtually unknown until the twentieth century. But now they're in every supermarket, and they're the stars in this chapter.

Boosting Beta-Carotene

You know when you see a food that's orange, it's probably high in beta-carotene, one of the most powerful antioxidants. While carrots hold first place for vegetables, both mangos and papayas are contenders in the fruit category.

Oranges are perhaps one of the best foods in this regard because the beta-carotene is balanced by such a high content of vitamin C. While other citrus fruits can't match up in beta-carotene content, they all add nutrients to these luscious libations.

Mixed Citrus

4 oranges

1 grapefruit

¼ lime

2 TB. honey

2 orange slices for garnish (optional)

Serves 2

Prep time:
less than 10 minutes

Each serving:
245 calories
5 calories from fat
0.5 g fat
0 g saturated fat
4 g protein
63 g carbohydrates

1. Peel and quarter oranges. Peel grapefruit and cut into sixths. Peel lime.

2. Push oranges, grapefruit, and lime through the juicer, and process until juiced. Pour juice into two glasses, add 1 tablespoon of honey to each, and stir well.

3. Serve immediately, garnished with orange slices if desired.

Variation: To pulp this recipe in a blender or food processor fitted with a steel blade, remove seeds from oranges, grapefruit, and lime, and cut all ingredients into pieces no larger than 1 inch.

Juicy Jive

Another benefit of juicing is having all the materials to make candied citrus peel. Cut the peel into ¼-inch strips and simmer in water for 20 minutes. Then drain and cook it with 1 cup of granulated sugar and ½ cup of water until it's soft. Remove it from the pan with a slotted spoon, and you've got delicious candy or an addition to baked goods.

Sparkling Citrus Juice

3 oranges

¼ lemon

¼ lime

¼ pineapple

½ cup sparkling mineral water

2 orange slices for garnish (optional)

Serves 2
Prep time:
less than 10 minutes
Each serving:
129 calories
0 calories from fat
0 g fat
0 g saturated fat
2 g protein
129 g carbohydrates

1. Peel and quarter oranges. Peel lemon and lime. Cut pineapple off rind and into 2-inch cubes.

2. Push oranges, lemon, lime, and pineapple through the juicer, and process until juiced. Pour juice into two glasses, and stir ¼ cup sparkling water into each glass.

3. Serve immediately, garnished with orange slices if desired.

Variation: To pulp this recipe in a blender or food processor fitted with a steel blade, remove seeds from oranges, lemon, and lime, and cut all ingredients into pieces no larger than 1 inch.

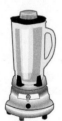

Wrong Spin!

A great deal of variation exists amongst sparkling waters and seltzers. What's important is to make sure the water is naturally sparkling from a mineral spring. Otherwise it can be just artificially carbonated tap water without any nutritional benefits.

Gingered Orange and Banana

4 oranges

2 bananas

4 TB. sliced fresh ginger

½ cup silken tofu

2 orange slices for garnish (optional)

Serves 2

Prep time:
less than 10 minutes

Each serving:
265 calories
9 calories from fat
1 g fat
0 g saturated fat
5 g protein
65 g carbohydrates

1. Peel oranges and quarter. Peel and slice bananas.

2. Push oranges and ginger through the juicer, and process until juiced. Pour juice into a blender, and add bananas and *tofu*. Blend for 30 seconds, and pour juice into two glasses.

3. Serve immediately, garnished with orange slices if desired.

Variation: To pulp this recipe in a blender or food processor fitted with a steel blade, remove seeds from oranges, peel ginger, and cut all ingredients into pieces no larger than 1 inch. If using a blender or food processor, add bananas and tofu along with other ingredients.

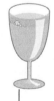

Liquid Lingo

Tofu is a custard-like substance made from the iron-rich liquid that comes from cooking ground soybeans. The process is similar to cheese making because the curds are drained and pressed, and the texture can range from silken to firm depending on how much whey is extracted. Silken is best for drinks like juices and smoothies.

Orange, Mango, and Lime

3 oranges

1 mango

2 celery ribs

¼ lime

2 orange slices for garnish (optional)

Serves 2
Prep time: less than 10 minutes
Each serving: 172 calories 9 calories from fat 1 g fat 0 g saturated fat 3 g protein 44 g carbohydrates

1. Peel oranges and cut into quarters. Peel mango and cut into 2-inch pieces. Rinse celery and cut into 2-inch lengths. Peel lime.

2. Push oranges, mango, celery, and lime through the juicer, and process until juiced. Stir well and pour juice into two glasses.

3. Serve immediately, garnished with orange slices if desired.

Variation: To pulp this recipe in a blender or food processor fitted with a steel blade, remove seeds from oranges and lime, and cut all ingredients into pieces no larger than 1 inch.

Pulp Tidbits

While scurvy, the disease resulting from too little vitamin C in the diet, was cured centuries ago, other medicinal benefits of vitamin C continue to grow. Nobel Prize–winning biochemist Linus Pauling was a strong advocate of large doses of vitamin C as a way to combat the common cold, and he collaborated with British cancer surgeon Ewan Cameron to publish a theory on vitamin C's value in fighting cancer as well.

Grapefruit, Orange, and Pineapple

2 grapefruit

2 oranges

¼ pineapple

¼ lemon

2 pineapple spears for garnish (optional)

Serves 2
Prep time: less than 10 minutes
Each serving: 236 calories 9 calories from fat 1 g fat 0 saturated fat 4 g protein 60 g carbohydrates

1. Peel grapefruit and cut into sixths. Peel oranges and quarter. Cut pineapple off rind and into 2-inch cubes. Peel lemon.

2. Push grapefruit, oranges, pineapple, and lemon through the juicer, and process until juiced. Stir well and pour juice into two glasses.

3. Serve immediately, garnished with pineapple spears if desired.

Variation: To pulp this recipe in a blender or food processor fitted with a steel blade, remove seeds from grapefruit, oranges, and lemon, and cut all ingredients into pieces no larger than 1 inch.

Pulp Tidbits

The English word pineapple evolved because of the fruit's resemblance to a pine cone rather than anything to do with its flavor or color. The Tupi word for the fruit was *anana*, which means "excellent fruit." Hummingbirds, which are native to the tropics, are the natural pollinators for pineapple.

Tangerine, Apple, and Pomegranate

4 tangerines

2 apples

1 pomegranate

1 cucumber

2 tangerine segments for garnish (optional)

Serves 2
Prep time:
less than 10 minutes
Each serving:
239 calories
9 calories from fat
1 g fat
0 g saturated fat
3 g protein
61 g carbohydrates

1. Peel tangerines and cut into quarters. Rinse apples and cut into sixths. Break pomegranate apart, pull out red pulp, and discard rind. Rinse cucumber and cut into 2-inch lengths.

2. Push tangerines, apples, pomegranate, and cucumber through the juicer, and process until juiced. Stir well and pour juice into two glasses.

3. Serve immediately, garnished with tangerine segments if desired.

Variation: To pulp this recipe in a blender or food processor fitted with a steel blade, remove seeds from tangerines if necessary, core apples, and cut all ingredients into pieces no larger than 1 inch. Drain mixture to remove pomegranate seeds.

Juicy Jive

While tangerines have a distinctive flavor, you can always substitute oranges for them in any juicing recipe. For every four tangerines use three oranges.

Minted Pineapple and Papaya

½ large papaya or 2 small papayas

¼ pineapple

1 cup green grapes

1 sprig mint

¼ lime

2 mint sprigs for garnish (optional)

Serves 2
Prep time:
less than 10 minutes
Each serving:
205 calories
9 calories from fat
1 g fat
0 g saturated fat
3 g protein
53 g carbohydrates

1. Peel papaya, discard seeds, and cut into 2-inch cubes. Cut pineapple off rind and into 2-inch cubes. Rinse grapes and mint. Peel lime.

2. Push papaya, pineapple, grapes, mint, and lime through the juicer, and process until juiced. Stir well and pour juice into two glasses.

3. Serve immediately, garnished with mint sprigs if desired.

Variation: To pulp this recipe in a blender or food processor fitted with a steel blade, remove seeds from lime and cut all ingredients into pieces no larger than 1 inch.

Juicy Jive

Two very distinct species of papaya are available in American supermarkets today. They both taste delicious, but their size is markedly different. Small papayas are the same size as a mango, while the large ones are about a foot long. That's why recipes in this book give two measurements for papaya.

Pineapple, Kiwi, and Strawberry

¼ pineapple

1 pint strawberries

3 kiwi

2 celery ribs

2 pineapple spears for garnish (optional)

Serves 2
Prep time: less than 10 minutes
Each serving: 170 calories 9 calories from fat 1 g fat 0 g saturated fat 3 g protein 42 g carbohydrates

1. Cut pineapple off rind and into 2-inch cubes. Rinse strawberries and kiwi. Rinse celery and cut into 2-inch lengths.

2. Push pineapple, strawberries, kiwi, and celery through the juicer, and process until juiced. Stir well and pour juice into two glasses.

3. Serve immediately, garnished with pineapple spears if desired.

Variation: To pulp this recipe in a blender or food processor fitted with a steel blade, cut tops off strawberries, peel kiwis, and cut all ingredients into pieces no larger than 1 inch.

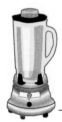

Wrong Spin!

Don't use a juice containing pineapple if you want to turn the juice into a gelatin dessert. Pineapple contains an enzyme, bromelian, that makes gelatin impossible to thicken.

Mango, Orange, and Banana

2 mangoes

2 oranges

¼ lime

2 bananas

2 mango spears for garnish (optional)

Serves 2
Prep time: less than 10 minutes
Each serving: 312 calories 9 calories from fat 1 g fat 0 g saturated fat 4 g protein 81 g carbohydrates

1. Peel mangoes, discard stones, and cut fruit into 2-inch cubes. Peel oranges and cut into quarters. Peel lime. Peel and slice bananas.

2. Push mangoes, oranges, and lime through the juicer, and process until juiced. Pour juice into a blender and add bananas. Blend for 30 seconds, and pour juice into two glasses.

3. Serve immediately, garnished with mango spears if desired.

Variation: To pulp this recipe in a blender or food processor fitted with a steel blade, remove seeds from oranges and lime and cut all ingredients into pieces no larger than 1 inch. If using a blender or food processor, add bananas along with other ingredients.

Juicy Jive

Bananas give juices a luscious thick texture, but there's a reason why they are added in a blender rather than put through the juicer. They don't contain that much juice, and it's really the banana pulp that you're after to add its flavor.

Spiced Papaya, Pineapple, and Citrus

½ large papaya or 2 small papayas

¼ pineapple

2 oranges

1 grapefruit

¼ tsp. ground cinnamon

2 papaya spears for garnish (optional)

Serves 2
Prep time:
less than 10 minutes
Each serving:
268 calories
9 calories from fat
1 g fat
0 g saturated fat
4 g protein
68 g carbohydrates

1. Peel papaya, discard seeds, and cut fruit into 2-inch cubes. Cut pineapple off rind and into 2-inch cubes. Peel oranges and cut into quarters. Peel grapefruit and cut into sixths.

2. Push papaya, pineapple, oranges, and grapefruit through the juicer, and process until juiced. Pour juice into two glasses, and stir ⅛ teaspoon *cinnamon* into each.

3. Serve immediately, garnished with papaya spears if desired.

Variation: To pulp this recipe in a blender or food processor fitted with a steel blade, discard seeds from papaya, remove seeds from oranges and grapefruit, and cut all ingredients into pieces no larger than 1 inch. If using a blender or food processor, add cinnamon along with other ingredients.

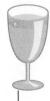

Liquid Lingo

Cinnamon is the inner bark of a tropical evergreen tree that's harvested during the rainy season and then allowed to dry. At that time it's sold ground or as sticks. What we call cinnamon is cassia cinnamon, and there's also a Ceylon cinnamon that is less pungent.

Kiwi, Guava, and Citrus

4 oranges

6 kiwi

4 guava

¼ lemon

2 orange slices for garnish (optional)

Serves 2
Prep time: less than 10 minutes
Each serving: 391 calories 27 calories from fat 3 g fat 0.5 g saturated fat 9 g protein 92 g carbohydrates

1. Peel and quarter oranges. Rinse kiwis and *guava*. Peel lemon.

2. Push oranges, kiwi, guava, and lemon through the juicer, and process until juiced. Stir well and pour juice into two glasses.

3. Serve immediately, garnished with orange slices if desired.

Variation: To pulp this recipe in a blender or food processor fitted with a steel blade, discard seeds from oranges and lemon, peel kiwi and guava, and cut all ingredients into pieces no larger than 1 inch.

Liquid Lingo

Guava is a fragrant tropical fruit that is oval and can range in size from an egg to a medium apple. The thin skin can be any color from yellow to purple black, and the aromatic sweet flesh is usually bright red. Allow green ones to ripen at room temperature.

Mixed Tropical Fruit

¼ large papaya or 1 small papaya

¼ pineapple

1 orange

1 mango

¼ lime

2 pineapple spears for garnish (optional)

Serves 2
Prep time:
less than 10 minutes
Each serving:
208 calories
9 calories from fat
1 g fat
0 g saturated fat
3 g protein
54 g carbohydrates

1. Peel papaya, discard seeds, and cut fruit into 2-inch cubes. Cut pine-apple off rind and into 2-inch cubes. Peel orange and quarter. Peel mango, discard stone, and cut into 2-inch cubes. Peel lime.

2. Push papaya, pineapple, orange, mango, and lime through the juicer, and process until juiced. Stir well and pour juice into two glasses.

3. Serve immediately, garnished with pineapple spears if desired.

Variation: To pulp this recipe in a blender or food processor fitted with a steel blade, discard seeds from orange and lime and cut all ingredients into pieces no larger than 1 inch.

Juicy Jive

Save papaya skins and add them to marinades. Papaya is very high in papain, an enzyme that is the basis for many natural meat tenderizers. The papaya skin will not give marinated foods any flavor, but you'll have much more succulent meats.

Part 4

Lean and Luscious Libations

Juices go upscale and sophisticated with the chapters in this part. These recipes are really beverages rather than just juices.

In one chapter you'll find various healthful teas combined with fruits. These are a treat at any time and can become party punches. The second chapter in this part turns juices into cocktails with the optional inclusion of liquor or wine.

Chapter 14

Tea Party

In This Chapter

- ◆ Fruit juices mixed with black tea
- ◆ Delicate green tea drinks
- ◆ Party punches

Juices and beverages made with fresh juices are sociable drinks, and this chapter's recipes are perfect party fare. The basis for these refreshing drinks are different teas that you combine with various fruits, spices, and even a few vegetables.

Like all recipes in this book, these juices make two servings. But you can multiply them as many times as you'd like if you're filling a punch bowl.

Touting Tea

Tea is the most commonly consumed beverage in the world after water. This is good news, because tea offers important health benefits as well as hydration.

Green tea was the first tea studied for its cancer-fighting benefits. But recent studies indicate that any tea derived from the leaf of a warm-weather evergreen known as *Camellia sinensis* has similar properties. This includes all green, black, and red (oolong) teas. The leaves of this tree contain chemicals called *polyphenols*, which give tea its antioxidant punch. Herbal teas do not derive from this leaf and so do not have this particular health-promoting chemical.

The degree of processing determines whether a tea will be green, black, or red. Green teas are the least processed. They are simply steamed quickly before packaging. Black and red teas are partially dried, crushed, and fermented. The length of fermentation, which causes the leaves to blacken, determines whether the tea will be red or black.

> **Liquid Lingo**
>
> **Polyphenols** are anti-oxidants that help protect cells from the damage of free radicals, neutralize enzymes essential for tumor growth, and deactivate cancer promoters. They are now known to help prevent cancer, and they are tied to preventing heart disease.

Tea also has fluoride for strong teeth, virtually no calories, and half the amount of caffeine found in an equal size cup of coffee. The question hasn't been answered as to whether decaffeinated teas have the same polyphenols. Caffeine is a natural component of tea leaves. We do not yet know if removing caffeine also removes polyphenols.

Brewing Bravado

Centuries-old rituals go into brewing the perfect cup of tea, and every self-respecting native of either China or England would balk at the sight of a tea bag sitting in a cup.

The first step of this brewing process is to warm the tea pot with very hot water, and then drain it. Then place the loose tea into the empty pot, and pour water over it. The temperature of the water and the amount of time needed for the tea to brew varies with the type of tea:

- Green tea should *steep* in 200°F water for 2 to 3 minutes.

- Oolong tea should steep in 200°F water for 4 to 7 minutes.

- Black teas, such as Irish or English, should be brewed by water at a full boil and allowed to brew for 3 to 5 minutes.

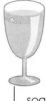

Liquid Lingo

Steep is the verb used when dry ingredients, such as tea leaves, herbs, or dried mushrooms, are soaked in hot liquid until the flavor of the ingredient is infused into the liquid.

The Herbal Alternative

A number of plants, both herbs and flowers, are dried and brewed into tea. Some of the more popular are chamomile, which many devotees say calms the nerves and lessens muscle cramps, and rosehip tea that's made from the berries formed by wild roses. Tea made from the petals of St. John's wort is touted as possibly relieving depression.

Rosemary, sage, thyme, ginger, and cinnamon are all used to infuse herbal teas. Herbal teas don't contain any caffeine, but they also don't have the same antioxidant benefits as green or black tea.

Black Tea, Orange, and Peach

3 ripe peaches

2 oranges

1 cup strongly brewed black tea, very chilled

¼ cup peach nectar

2 peach slices for garnish (optional)

Serves 2
Prep time: less than 10 minutes
Each serving:
139 calories
9 calories from fat
1 g fat
0 g saturated fat
3 g protein
35 g carbohydrates

1. Rinse peaches, discard stones, and cut into 2-inch pieces. Peel and quarter oranges.

2. Push peaches and oranges through the juicer, and process until juiced. Pour juice into two glasses. Stir ½ cup tea and ⅛ cup nectar into each glass.

3. Serve immediately, garnished with peach slices if desired.

Variation: To pulp this recipe in a blender or food processor fitted with a steel blade, remove seeds from oranges and cut all ingredients into pieces no larger than 1 inch. If using a blender or food processor, add tea and nectar along with other ingredients.

Pulp Tidbits

Cultivation of tea plants began in China more than 4,000 years ago but was kept a secret until the eighth century C.E. when the Japanese adopted it. Europeans didn't learn of tea until the seventeenth century, at which time the British spread its growing areas into India.

Black Tea, Raspberry, and Pineapple

¼ pineapple

1 (6-oz.) container raspberries

1 cup strongly brewed black tea, very chilled

2 TB. fruit-only raspberry preserves

2 pineapple spears for garnish (optional)

Serves 2
Prep time:
less than 10 minutes
Each serving:
149 calories
9 calories from fat
1 g fat
0 g saturated fat
2 g protein
37 g carbohydrates

1. Cut pineapple off rind and into 2-inch cubes. Rinse raspberries.

2. Push pineapple and raspberries through the juicer, and process until juiced. Pour juice into two glasses, and stir ½ cup tea and 1 tablespoon preserves into each glass.

3. Serve immediately, garnished with pineapple spears if desired.

Variation: To pulp this recipe in a blender or food processor fitted with a steel blade, cut pineapple into pieces no larger than 1 inch. If using a blender or food processor, add tea and preserves with other ingredients.

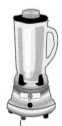

Wrong Spin!

Fruit-only preserves are not just made with the fruit listed on the label. Most of the time they are sweetened with apple juice concentrate. This concentrate is high in calories but they're not the "empty calories" contained in refined sugar.

Black Tea, Apple, and Pear

3 apples

2 pears

1 cup strongly brewed black tea, very chilled

2 apple wedges for garnish (optional)

Serves 2

Prep time:
less than 10 minutes

Each serving:
210 calories
9 calories from fat
1 g fat
0 g saturated fat
1 g protein
56 g carbohydrates

1. Rinse apples and cut into sixths. Rinse and quarter pears.

2. Push apples and pears through the juicer, and process until juiced. Pour juice into two glasses, and stir $\frac{1}{2}$ cup tea into each glass.

3. Serve immediately, garnished with apple slices if desired.

Variation: To pulp this recipe in a blender or food processor fitted with a steel blade, core apples and pears, and cut all ingredients into pieces no larger than 1 inch. If using a blender or food processor, add tea with other ingredients.

Juicy Jive

Like bananas, pears ripen better off the tree than they do on it. If you're in a hurry to ripen pears, place them in a plastic bag with a few apples. The apples let off a natural gas that hastens ripening.

Creamy Spiced Apple Chai

4 apples

½ fresh fennel bulb

2 TB. fresh ginger

½ cup strongly brewed black tea

½ cup soy milk

2 TB. firmly packed dark brown sugar

½ tsp. ground cinnamon

¼ tsp. ground allspice

2 apple wedges for garnish (optional)

Serves 2
Prep time: less than 10 minutes
Each serving: 257 calories 18 calories from fat 2 g fat 0 g saturated fat 4 g protein 62 g carbohydrates

1. Rinse apples and cut into sixths. Rinse fennel, trim stem end, and cut into 2-inch cubes.

2. Push apples, fennel, and ginger through the juicer, and process until juiced. Pour juice into two glasses, and stir ¼ cup tea, ¼ cup soy milk, 1 tablespoon brown sugar, ¼ teaspoon cinnamon, and ⅛ teaspoon allspice into each glass.

3. Serve immediately, garnished with apple wedges if desired.

Variation: To pulp this recipe in a blender or food processor fitted with a steel blade, core apples, peel ginger, and cut all ingredients into pieces no larger than 1 inch. If using a blender or food processor, add tea, soy milk, brown sugar, cinnamon, and allspice with other ingredients.

Pulp Tidbits

Chai, pronounced as a single syllable that rhymes with "pie," is a spiced tea and milk mixture of Indian origin. The spices used vary from region to region in India, but the faithful believe that drinking it aids digestion.

Green Tea, Mango, and Pineapple

2 mangoes

¼ pineapple

¼ lime

1 cup brewed green tea, very chilled

2 mango spears for garnish (optional)

Serves 2
Prep time: less than 10 minutes
Each serving: 175 calories 9 calories from fat 1 g fat 0 g saturated fat 1 g protein 46 g carbohydrates

1. Peel mangoes, discard stones, and cut into 2-inch cubes. Cut pineapple from rind and into 2-inch cubes. Peel lime.

2. Push mangoes and pineapple through the juicer, and process until juiced. Pour juice into two glasses, and stir ½ cup tea into each glass.

3. Serve immediately, garnished with mango spears if desired.

Variation: To pulp this recipe in a blender or food processor fitted with a steel blade, remove lime seeds and cut all ingredients into pieces no larger than 1 inch. If using a blender or food processor, add green tea with other ingredients.

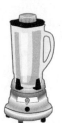

Wrong Spin!

One of the newcomers to the produce section is pre-peeled mangoes, and while they offer great convenience, you should pass them by. I've tried a few brands, and most of the mango was acidic and not ripe, plus many of the nutrients dissipate after peeling.

Green Tea and Citrus

3 oranges

1 grapefruit

¼ lime

3 TB. crystallized ginger

1 cup brewed green tea, very chilled

2 orange slices for garnish (optional)

Serves 2
Prep time: less than 10 minutes
Each serving: 176 calories 0 calories from fat 0 g fat 0 g saturated fat 3 g protein 45 g carbohydrates

1. Peel and quarter oranges. Peel grapefruit and cut into sixths. Peel lime.

2. Push oranges, grapefruit, and lime through the juicer, and process until juiced. Pour juice into a blender, and add *crystallized ginger* and green tea. Blend for 30 seconds, and pour juice into two glasses.

3. Serve immediately, garnished with orange slices if desired.

Variation: To pulp this recipe in a blender or food processor fitted with a steel blade, remove seeds from oranges, grapefruit, and lime, and cut all ingredients into pieces no larger than 1 inch. If using a blender or food processor, add ginger and tea with other ingredients.

Liquid Lingo

Crystallized ginger is fresh ginger that has been cooked in a sugar syrup and then coated with coarse sugar. It is a preserved form of ginger but has more fresh ginger taste than ground ginger.

Green Tea, Lychee, and Lime

½ lb. fresh lychee nuts

½ lime

1 cup brewed green tea, very chilled

2 lime wedges for garnish (optional)

Serves 2
Prep time:
less than 10 minutes
Each serving:
322 calories
9 calories from fat
1 g fat
0 saturated fat
4 g protein
83 g carbohydrates

1. Peel lychee nuts and discard pits. Peel lime.

2. Push lychee nuts and lime through the juicer, and process until juiced. Pour juice into two glasses, and stir ½ cup tea into each glass.

3. Serve immediately, garnished with lime wedges if desired.

Variation: To pulp this recipe in a blender or food processor fitted with a steel blade, remove lime seeds. If using a blender or food processor, add tea with other ingredients.

Juicy Jive

Fresh lychee nuts have an incredibly succulent flavor, but they are still difficult to find in most parts of the country. If you live near the Chinese section of any city, try the markets in those neighborhoods. They're far more likely to stock them.

Tropical Peppermint

1 mango

½ large papaya or 1 small papaya

2 oranges

¼ lime

1 cup brewed peppermint tea, very chilled

2 orange slices for garnish (optional)

Serves 2
Prep time: less than 10 minutes
Each serving: 196 calories 9 calories from fat 1 g fat 0 g saturated fat 3 g protein 50 g carbohydrates

1. Peel mango, discard seed, and cut into 2-inch pieces. Peel papaya, scrape out seeds, and cut into 2-inch pieces. Peel oranges and quarter. Peel lime.

2. Push mango, papaya, oranges, and lime through the juicer, and process until juiced. Pour juice into two glasses, and stir ½ cup tea into each glass.

3. Serve immediately, garnished with orange slices if desired.

Variation: To pulp this recipe in a blender or food processor fitted with a steel blade, remove seeds from oranges and lime and cut all ingredients into pieces no larger than 1 inch. If using a blender or food processor, add tea with other ingredients.

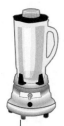

Wrong Spin!

The peppermint tea used in this recipe is an herbal tea made with dried peppermint leaves. Some packagers also have a peppermint-flavored black tea that is made with artificial peppermint flavoring. Be sure to buy the herbal tea.

Chamomile and Berries

1 pint strawberries

1 (6-oz.) container raspberries

1 apple

1 cup brewed chamomile tea, very chilled

2 strawberries for garnish (optional)

Serves 2
Prep time:
less than 10 minutes
Each serving:
131 calories
9 calories from fat
1 g fat
0 g saturated fat
2 g protein
32 g carbohydrates

1. Rinse strawberries and raspberries. Rinse apple and cut into sixths.

2. Push strawberries, raspberries, and apple through the juicer, and process until juiced. Pour the juice into two glasses, and stir ½ cup tea into each glass.

3. Serve immediately, garnished with strawberries if desired.

Variation: To pulp this recipe in a blender or food processor fitted with a steel blade, remove tops from strawberries, core apple, and cut all ingredients into pieces no larger than 1 inch. If using a blender or food processor, add tea with other ingredients.

Juicy Jive

If you want to freeze your berries and pulp this drink, then rinse them and remove the green tops of the strawberries before you freeze them.

Chapter 15

Juices with a Jolt

In This Chapter

- ◆ Juices to spike as cocktails
- ◆ Juices to blend with wines
- ◆ Juices to serve as "mock-tails"

Don't banish your juicer when you're entertaining. You won't believe the difference it makes as you create fresh juices to use as mixers for cocktails. And I give you recipes for these in this chapter. For teenagers and those who choose not to drink alcohol, these recipes also give ways to make your drinks taste like the real thing and still be safe for all to consume.

In addition to cocktails, this chapter contains a number of recipes for wine punches made with fresh fruits. You can serve any of these as a punch for a large group.

Nonalcoholic Alternatives

You can achieve the same sense of sophistication of enjoying a cocktail without adding alcohol to your bloodstream. As vodka has virtually no taste, just don't add it to any recipe. For rum, the other liquor specified in many of these recipes, a dash of rum extract adds a flavor that is similar.

With wines it's even easier to omit the alcohol. Many options are available for nonalcoholic wines, some of which are produced by famous wineries and have a delicious flavor. They're made from the same grape varietals used for the "hard stuff" and with a similar process as wine with one big difference—no alcohol is added for fermentation.

Another alternative is to use sparkling apple cider in place of non-alcoholic wine. Cider will add an additional layer of fruity taste to any recipe.

Bloody Mary

8 ripe tomatoes

¼ red bell pepper

1 celery rib

¼ lemon

2 TB. Worcestershire sauce

1 TB. prepared horseradish

2 tsp. soy sauce

½ to 1 tsp. hot red pepper sauce

2 to 3 oz. vodka (optional)

Ice cubes

2 celery sprigs for garnish (optional)

Serves 2
Prep time: less than 10 minutes
Each serving: 230 calories 18 calories from fat 2 g fat 0 g saturated fat 5 g protein 30 g carbohydrates

1. Rinse tomatoes and cut into quarters. Discard cap and seeds from bell pepper and cut into 2-inch pieces. Rinse celery and cut into 2-inch lengths. Peel lemon.

2. Push tomatoes, bell pepper, celery, and lemon through the juicer, and process until juiced. Pour juice into a pitcher, and add Worcestershire sauce, horseradish, soy sauce, hot pepper sauce, and vodka (if used). Stir well and pour juice into two glasses over ice cubes.

3. Serve immediately, garnished with celery sprigs if desired.

Variation: To pulp this recipe in a blender or food processor fitted with a steel blade, core tomatoes, peel lemon, and cut all ingredients into pieces no larger than 1 inch. If using a blender or food processor, add additional ingredients along with vegetables.

Pulp Tidbits

While it was popularized at the King Cole Bar at New York's St. Regis Hotel in the 1920s, the Bloody Mary was actually born in Paris at Harry's New York Bar. Ferdinand Petiot, the bartender, concocted it for some American clients. When he was hired by the St. Regis, he brought the drink with him.

Jalapeño Mary

8 ripe tomatoes

1 carrot

½ red bell pepper

1 jalapeño or serrano chili pepper

¼ lime

1 garlic clove

1 TB. Worcestershire sauce

2 tsp. Cajun seasoning

2 to 3 oz. vodka (optional)

Ice cubes

2 red pepper slices for garnish (optional)

Serves 2
Prep time: less than 10 minutes
Each serving: 246 calories 18 calories from fat 2 g fat 0 g saturated fat 5 g protein 34 g carbohydrates

1. Rinse tomatoes and quarter. Scrub carrot, discard tops, and cut into 2-inch lengths. Rinse red pepper and chili pepper, and discard cap and seeds. Peel lime.

2. Push tomatoes, carrot, bell pepper, chili pepper, lime, and garlic clove through the juicer, and process until juiced. Pour juice into a pitcher and add Worcestershire sauce, *Cajun seasoning*, and vodka (if used). Stir well and pour juice into two glasses over ice cubes.

3. Serve immediately, garnished with red pepper slices if desired.

Variation: To pulp this recipe in a blender or food processor fitted with a steel blade, remove seeds from lime, peel garlic, and cut all ingredients into pieces no larger than 1 inch. If using a blender or food processor, add Worcestershire sauce, Cajun seasoning, and vodka along with other ingredients.

Liquid Lingo

Cajun seasoning is a newcomer to the pre-mixed herb and spice blends. There is no one definition of the blend, although all are boldly flavored. Most contain onion, garlic, paprika, cayenne, and thyme.

Spicy Carrot Cocktail

3 carrots

3 tomatoes

2 celery ribs

$\frac{1}{2}$ red bell pepper

1 jalapeño or serrano chili

$\frac{1}{4}$ lemon

2 to 3 oz. vodka (optional)

2 tsp. ground cumin

Ice cubes

2 carrot sticks for garnish (optional)

Serves 2
Prep time: less than 10 minutes
Each serving: 203 calories 9 calories from fat 1 g fat 0 g saturated fat 3.5 g protein 23 g carbohydrates

1. Scrub carrots, discard tops, and cut into 2-inch lengths. Rinse tomatoes and cut into quarters. Rinse celery and cut into 2-inch lengths. Rinse bell pepper and jalapeño pepper, and discard cap and seeds. Peel lemon.

2. Push carrots, tomatoes, celery, bell pepper, jalapeño pepper, and lemon through the juicer, and process until juiced. Pour juice over ice cubes into two glasses, and stir 1 to $1\frac{1}{2}$ ounces vodka (if used) and 1 teaspoon ground cumin into each.

3. Serve immediately, garnished with carrot sticks if desired.

Variation: To pulp this recipe in a blender or food processor fitted with a steel blade, core tomatoes, remove lemon seeds, and cut all ingredients into pieces no larger than 1 inch. If using a blender or food processor, add vodka and cumin along with other ingredients.

Juicy Jive

It's common to see jalapeño and serrano chilies given as recipe options in the same quantity, although serrano peppers are much smaller. They are also much hotter, so the larger jalapeño and the small serrano produce the same amount of heat.

Cape Cod Cocktail

2 grapefruit

1 orange

½ cup fresh cranberries

¼ cup simple syrup

2 to 3 oz. vodka (optional)

Ice cubes

2 grapefruit sections for garnish (optional)

Serves 2
Prep time:
less than 10 minutes
Each serving:
296 calories
0 calories from fat
0 g fat
0 g saturated fat
3 g protein
51 g carbohydrates

1. Peel grapefruit and cut into sixths. Peel orange and cut into quarters. Rinse cranberries.

2. Push grapefruit, orange, and cranberries through the juicer, and process until juiced. Pour juice into two glasses, and stir ⅛ cup *simple syrup* and 1 to 1½ ounces vodka (if used) into each. Add ice cubes.

3. Serve immediately, garnished with grapefruit sections if desired.

Variation: To pulp this recipe in a blender or food processor fitted with a steel blade, remove seeds from grapefruit and orange and cut all ingredients into pieces no larger than 1 inch. If using a blender or food processor, add simple syrup and vodka (if used) along with other ingredients.

Liquid Lingo

Simple syrup is used to sweeten many drinks. It's a combination of two parts granulated sugar to one part water that is heated until the liquid is clear and the sugar is dissolved.

Piña Colada

½ pineapple

¼ lime

⅓ cup cream of coconut

2 to 3 oz. light rum or ¼ tsp. rum extract mixed with ¼ cup cold water

½ cup ice cubes

2 pineapple spears for garnish (optional)

Serves 2
Prep time:
less than 10 minutes
Each serving:
306 calories
126 calories from fat
14 g fat
12 g saturated fat
2 g protein
24 g carbohydrates

1. Cut pineapple off rind and into 2-inch cubes. Peel lime.

2. Push pineapple and lime through the juicer, and process until juiced. Pour juice into a blender, and add cream of coconut, rum, and ice cubes. Blend for 30 seconds, and pour juice into two glasses.

3. Serve immediately, garnished with pineapple spears if desired.

Variation: To pulp this recipe in a blender or food processor fitted with a steel blade, remove seeds from lime and cut all ingredients into pieces no larger than 1 inch. If using a blender or food processor, add cream of coconut, rum, and ice along with other ingredients.

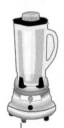

Wrong Spin! _____

Don't confuse cream of coconut with coconut milk or its richer cousin, coconut cream. Cream of coconut is highly sweetened and thick. Always stir it before adding it to a recipe as it tends to separate.

Strawberry Margarita

2 pints strawberries

½ lime

2 to 3 oz. tequila or ¼ tsp. rum extract mixed with ¼ cup cold water

1 oz. triple sec or other clear orange liqueur (optional)

1 cup crushed ice

2 strawberries for garnish (optional)

Serves 2
Prep time: less than 10 minutes
Each serving: 238 calories 9 calories from fat 1 g fat 0 g saturated fat 2 g protein 29 g carbohydrates

1. Rinse strawberries and discard tops. Peel lime.

2. Push strawberries and lime through the juicer, and process until juiced. Pour juice into a blender and add *tequila*, triple sec (if used), and ice. Blend for 30 seconds, and pour juice into two glasses.

3. Serve immediately, garnished with strawberries if desired.

Variation: To pulp this recipe in a blender or food processor fitted with a steel blade, cut tops off strawberries, remove seeds from lime, and cut all ingredients into pieces no larger than 1 inch. If using a blender or food processor, add tequila, tripe sec (if used), and ice along with other ingredients.

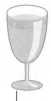

Liquid Lingo

Tequila is a clear or light yellow colored liquor made by distilling the sweet sap of the Mexican agave plant. It originated in Tequila, Mexico, which is how it got its name, and it's been imported into the United States since the mid-nineteenth century.

Mango Daiquiri

2 mangoes

1 lime

¼ cup simple syrup

2 to 3 oz. light rum or ¼ tsp. rum extract mixed with ¼ cup cold water

1 cup crushed ice

2 lime wedges for garnish (optional)

Serves 2
Prep time: less than 10 minutes
Each serving: 289 calories 9 calories from fat 1 g fat 0 g saturated fat 1 g protein 51 g carbohydrates

1. Peel mangoes, discard seeds, and cut into 2-inch cubes. Peel lime.

2. Push mangoes and lime through the juicer, and process until juiced. Pour juice into a blender, and add simple syrup, rum, and ice. Blend for 30 seconds, and pour juice into two glasses.

3. Serve immediately, garnished with lime wedges if desired.

Variation: To pulp this recipe in a blender or food processor fitted with a steel blade, cut all ingredients into pieces no larger than 1 inch. If using a blender or food processor, add simple syrup, rum or rum extract mixture, and ice along with other ingredients.

Juicy Jive

There are nifty ways to dress up these cocktail juices. Use a stemmed wine glass or a margarita glass, and dip the rim into water and then into granulated sugar or sea salt. You'll have a dramatic presentation and an ingredient to add its character.

Sangria

2 oranges

½ pt. strawberries

¼ lemon

¼ lime

1 cup red wine or nonalcoholic red wine

Ice cubes

2 orange slices for garnish (optional)

Serves 2
Prep time:
less than 10 minutes
Each serving:
193 calories
0 calories from fat
0 g fat
0 g saturated fat
2 g protein
26.5 g carbohydrates

1. Peel oranges and cut into quarters. Rinse strawberries and remove tops. Peel lemon and lime.

2. Push oranges, strawberries, lemon, and lime through the juicer, and process until juiced. Pour juice into two large glasses, and stir ½ cup wine into each. Add ice cubes.

3. Serve immediately, garnished with orange slices if desired.

Variation: To pulp this recipe in a blender or food processor fitted with a steel blade, remove seeds from oranges, lemon, and lime, cut tops off strawberries, and cut all ingredients into pieces no larger than 1 inch.

Juicy Jive

You can also make this drink with white wine, and add any fruit-flavored liqueur such as triple sec (orange flavor), crème de cassis (black currant flavor), or Chambord (raspberry flavor).

Sparkling Pineapple Sangria

¼ ripe pineapple

2 oranges

¼ lime

⅔ cup very chilled sparkling wine or non-alcoholic sparkling wine

2 to 3 oz. light rum (optional)

2 pineapple spears for garnish (optional)

Serves 2
Prep time: less than 10 minutes
Each serving: 275 calories 0 calories from fat 0 g fat 0 g saturated fat 2 g protein 31 g carbohydrates

1. Cut pineapple off rind and into 2-inch cubes. Peel and quarter oranges. Peel lime.

2. Push pineapple, oranges, and lime through the juicer, and process until juiced. Pour juice into two large glasses. Stir ⅓ cup *sparkling wine* into each glass.

3. Serve immediately, garnished with pineapple spears if desired.

Variation: To pulp this recipe in a blender or food processor fitted with a steel blade, remove seeds from oranges and lime, and cut all ingredients into pieces no larger than 1-inch.

Liquid Lingo

Sparkling wine is the overall term used to describe wine that contains bubbles of carbon dioxide. It is produced by the French *méthode champenoise* during which the wine is given a second fermentation that takes place in the bottle, which creates the carbon dioxide. You should only use the term Champagne for those sparkling wines from that specific region of France.

Sparkling Spiced Papaya and Banana Sangria

½ large papaya or 2 small papayas

1 orange

¼ lime

1 banana

⅔ cup very chilled sparkling wine or non-alcoholic sparkling wine

¼ tsp. ground cinnamon

2 orange slices for garnish (optional)

Serves 2
Prep time: less than 10 minutes
Each serving: 275 calories 9 calories from fat 1 g fat 0 g saturated fat 3 g protein 55 g carbohydrates

1. Peel papaya, discard seeds, and cut into 2-inch cubes. Peel and quarter orange. Peel lime. Peel and slice banana.

2. Push papaya, orange, and lime through the juicer, and process until juiced. Pour juice into a blender, and add banana, sparkling wine, and cinnamon. Blend for 30 seconds, and pour juice into two glasses.

3. Serve immediately, garnished with orange slices if desired.

Variation: To pulp this recipe in a blender or food processor fitted with a steel blade, remove seeds from orange and lime and cut all ingredients into pieces no larger than 1 inch. If using a blender or food processor, add banana, sparkling wine, and cinnamon along with other ingredients.

Juicy Jive

While adding ice cubes to wine-based sangria is fine, it causes the bubbles to instantly disappear from sparkling wine. That's why the wine should be very well chilled; it also helps if the fruits are chilled, too.

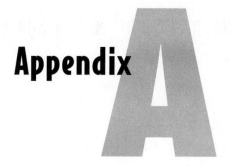

Appendix A

Glossary

acidophilus A friendly bacteria used to thicken yogurt.

allspice Named for its flavor echoes of several spices (cinnamon, cloves, nutmeg), allspice is used in many desserts and in rich marinades and stews.

almonds Mild, sweet, and crunchy nuts that combine nicely with creamy and sweet food items.

Anaheim peppers Long, light green peppers with only a hint of hotness used frequently for stuffing.

artichoke hearts The center part of the artichoke flower, often found canned in grocery stores and used as a stand-alone vegetable dish or as a flavorful base for appetizers or main courses.

arugula A spicy-peppery garden plant with leaves that resemble a dandelion and have a distinctive—and very sharp—flavor.

balsamic vinegar Vinegar produced primarily in Italy from a specific type of grape and aged in wood barrels. It is heavier, darker, and sweeter than most vinegars.

basil A flavorful, almost sweet, resinous herb delicious with tomatoes and used in all kinds of Italian and Mediterranean-style dishes.

Belgian endive A plant that resembles a small, elongated, tightly packed head of romaine lettuce. The thick, crunchy leaves can be broken off and used with dips and spreads.

black pepper A biting and pungent seasoning, freshly ground pepper is a must for many dishes and adds an extra level of flavor and taste.

blend To completely mix something, usually with a blender or food processor, more slowly than beating.

bok choy (also **Chinese cabbage**) A member of the cabbage family with thick stems, crisp texture, and fresh flavor. It is perfect for stir-frying.

caraway A distinctive spicy seed used for bread, pork, cheese, and cabbage dishes. It is known to reduce stomach upset, which is why it is often paired with, for example, sauerkraut.

carbohydrate A nutritional component found in starches, sugars, fruits, and vegetables that causes a rise in blood glucose levels. Carbohydrates supply energy and many important nutrients, including vitamins, minerals, and antioxidants.

cardamom An intense, sweet-smelling spice, common to Indian cooking, used in baking and coffee.

cayenne A fiery spice made from (hot) chili peppers, especially the cayenne chili, a slender, red, and very hot pepper.

chickpeas (also **garbanzo beans**) A yellow-gold, roundish bean that's the base ingredient in hummus. Chickpeas are high in fiber and low in fat, making this a delicious and healthful component of many appetizers and main dishes.

chilis (also **chiles**) Any one of many different "hot" peppers, ranging in intensity from the relatively mild ancho pepper to the blisteringly hot habañero.

chili powder A seasoning blend that includes chili pepper, cumin, garlic, and oregano. Proportions vary among different versions, but all offer a warm, rich flavor.

Chinese five-spice powder A seasoning blend of cinnamon, anise, ginger, fennel, and pepper.

chives   A member of the onion family, chives grow in bunches of long leaves that resemble tall grass or the green tops of onions. Chives provide a light onion flavor to any dish. They're very easy to grow and are often grown in gardens.

chop   To cut into pieces, usually qualified by an adverb such as "*coarsely* chopped," or by a size measurement such as "chopped into ½-inch pieces." "Finely chopped" is much closer to mince.

cider vinegar   A mild vinegar distilled from apple cider.

cilantro   A member of the parsley family used in Mexican cooking and some Asian dishes. Cilantro is what gives some salsas their unique flavor. Use in moderation, as the flavor can overwhelm. The seed of the cilantro is the spice coriander.

cinnamon   A sweet, rich, aromatic spice commonly used in baking or desserts. Cinnamon can also be used for delicious and interesting entrées.

clove   A sweet, strong, almost wintergreen-flavored spice used in baking and with meats such as ham.

complete protein   A food that contains all the essential amino acids necessary for the growth of cells.

core   As a noun the woody center of fruits such as apples and pears, and as a verb to remove that part of the fruit.

coriander   A rich, warm, spicy seed used in all types of recipes, from African to South American, from entrées to desserts.

crudités   Fresh vegetables served as an appetizer, often all together on one tray.

crystallized ginger   Fresh ginger that has been preserved by cooking it in a sugar syrup.

cumin   A fiery, smoky-tasting spice popular in Middle-Eastern, Mexican, and Indian dishes. Cumin is a seed; ground cumin seed is the most common form of the spice used in cooking.

curry   A general term referring to rich, spicy, Indian-style sauces and the dishes prepared with them. A curry will use curry powder as its base seasoning.

curry powder   A ground blend of spices used as a basis for curry and a huge range of other Indian-influenced dishes. All blends are rich and flavorful. Some, such as Vindaloo and Madras, are notably hotter than others. Common ingredients include hot pepper, nutmeg, cumin, cinnamon, pepper, and turmeric. Some curry can also be found in paste form.

dash   A few drops, usually of a liquid, released by a quick shake of, for example, a bottle of hot sauce.

dice   To cut into small cubes about ¼-inch square.

dietary minerals   Chemical elements required by all living organisms that come from the makeup of the soil.

Dijon mustard   Hearty, spicy mustard made in the style of the Dijon region of France.

dill   A unique herb that is perfect for eggs, salmon, cheese dishes, and, of course, vegetables (pickles!).

dry-packed   The way fruit is described when it's frozen in individual pieces without additional sugar or in a syrup.

drizzle   To lightly sprinkle drops of a liquid over food. Drizzling is often the finishing touch to a dish.

extra-virgin olive oil   *See* olive oil.

fennel   In seed form, a fragrant, licorice-tasting herb. The bulbs have a much milder flavor and a celery-like crunch and are used as a vegetable in salads or cooked recipes.

floret   The flower or bud end of broccoli or cauliflower.

fraises du bois   Tiny French strawberries with intense flavor.

fructose   Sugar naturally found in fruit, slightly sweeter than table sugar.

garlic   A member of the onion family, a pungent and flavorful element in many savory dishes. A garlic bulb, the form in which garlic is often sold, contains multiple cloves. Each clove, when chopped, provides about 1 teaspoon garlic. Most recipes call for cloves or chopped garlic by the teaspoon.

garnish   An embellishment not vital to the dish but added to enhance visual appeal.

ginger   Available in fresh root or dried, ground form, ginger adds a pungent, sweet, and spicy quality to a dish. It is a very popular element of many Asian and Indian dishes, among others.

glucose   The simplest natural sugar.

granita   The Italian word for ice used to describe granular mixtures served like sorbet.

grate   To shave into tiny pieces using a sharp rasp or grater.

grind   To reduce a large, hard substance, often a seasoning such as peppercorns, to the consistency of sand.

guava   A fragrant tropical fruit that is oval and can range in size from an egg to a medium apple.

hearts of palm   Firm, elongated, off-white cylinders from the inside of a palm tree stem tip. They are delicious in many recipes.

herbes de Provence   A seasoning mix including basil, fennel, marjoram, rosemary, sage, and thyme, common in the south of France.

hoisin sauce   A soybean-based thick sauce with a sweet and spicy flavor used in Chinese cooking.

horseradish   A sharp, spicy root that forms the flavor base in many condiments from cocktail sauce to sharp mustards. It is a natural match with roast beef. The form generally found in grocery stores is prepared horseradish, which contains vinegar and oil, among other ingredients. Use pure horseradish much more sparingly than the prepared version, or try cutting it with sour cream.

infusion   A liquid in which flavorful ingredients such as herbs have been soaked or steeped to extract that flavor into the liquid.

julienne   A French word meaning "to slice into very thin pieces."

kale   A vegetable belonging to the cabbage family that is mild in flavor and grows in bunches rather than as a head.

key limes   Very small limes grown primarily in Florida known for their tart taste.

kosher salt A coarse-grained salt made without any additives or iodine, used by many cooks because it does not impart a chemical flavor.

lychee A sweet and juicy fruit from China covered with a rough, bright red shell.

marjoram A sweet herb, a cousin of and similar to oregano, popular in Greek, Spanish, and Italian dishes.

mesclun Mixed salad greens, usually containing lettuce and assorted greens such as arugula, cress, endive, and others.

mince To cut into very small pieces smaller than diced pieces, about $1/8$ inch or smaller.

mold A decorative, shaped metal pan in which contents, such as mousse or gelatin, set up and take the shape of the pan.

mull (or **mulled**) To heat a liquid with the addition of spices and sometimes sweeteners.

nutmeg A sweet, fragrant, musky spice used primarily in baking.

nutrients Any elements needed by the body for metabolism, growth, or proper functioning.

olive oil A fragrant liquid produced by crushing or pressing olives. Extra-virgin olive oil is the oil produced from the first pressing of a batch of olives; oil is also produced from other pressings after the first. Extra-virgin olive oil is generally considered the most flavorful and highest quality and is the type you want to use when your focus is on the oil itself.

oregano A fragrant, slightly astringent herb used in Greek, Spanish, and Italian dishes.

oxidation The browning of fruit flesh that happens over time and with exposure to air. If you need to cut apples in advance, minimize oxidation by rubbing the cut surfaces with a lemon half. Oxidation also affects wine, which is why the taste changes over time after a bottle is opened.

parsley A fresh-tasting green leafy herb used to add color and interest to just about any savory dish. Often used as a garnish just before serving.

peppercorns Large, round, dried berries that are ground to produce pepper.

pesto A thick spread or sauce made with fresh basil leaves, garlic, olive oil, pine nuts, and Parmesan cheese. Some newer versions are made with other herbs. Pesto can be made at home or purchased in a grocery store and used on anything from appetizers to pasta and other main dishes.

pinch An unscientific measurement term that refers to the amount of an ingredient—typically a dry, granular substance such as an herb or seasoning—you can hold between your finger and thumb.

pine nuts Tiny nuts, called *piñon* in Spanish and *pignoli* in Italian, found inside the pine cones of various species of evergreen and used in Mexican and Italian cooking.

polyphenols Antioxidants found in all leaf tea.

purée To reduce a food to a thick, creamy texture, usually using a blender or food processor.

reserve To hold a specified ingredient for another use later in the recipe.

rhizome An underground part of the stem of a plant such as ginger.

rosemary A pungent, sweet herb used with chicken, pork, fish, and especially lamb. A little of it goes a long way.

saffron A famous spice made from the stamens of crocus flowers. Saffron lends a dramatic yellow color and distinctive flavor to a dish. Only a tiny amount needs to be used, which is good because saffron is very expensive.

sage An herb with a musty yet fruity, lemon-rind scent and "sunny" flavor. It is a terrific addition to many dishes.

salsa A style of mixing fresh vegetables and/or fresh fruit in a coarse chop. Salsa can be spicy or not, fruit-based or not, and served as a starter on its own (with chips, for example) or as a companion to a main course.

savory A popular herb with a fresh, woody taste.

shallot   A member of the onion family that grows in a bulb somewhat like garlic and has a milder onion flavor. When a recipe calls for shallot, use the entire bulb. (They might or might not have cloves.)

simple syrup   A mixture of two parts granulated sugar to one part water heated until the sugar dissolves.

slice   To cut into thin pieces.

soy milk   An iron-rich liquid made by pressing soybeans that are ground and cooked.

sparkling wine   The overall term used to describe wine that contains bubbles of carbon dioxide, the most famous being Champagne.

steep   To let dry ingredients sit in hot water until the flavor infuses into the liquid, such as tea leaves into tea, or until the food softens, such as dried mushrooms.

tahini   A paste made from sesame seeds that is used to flavor many Middle Eastern recipes, especially baba ghanoush and hummus.

tamari   A sauce made from soybeans similar to soy sauce but thicker and with a flavor that is more mellow.

tarragon   A sweet, rich-smelling herb perfect with seafood, vegetables (especially asparagus), chicken, and pork.

tequila   A Mexican liquor made by distilling the sap of the agave plant.

thyme   A minty, zesty herb whose leaves are used in a wide range of recipes.

tofu   A cheeselike substance made from soybeans and soy milk. Flavorful and nutritious, tofu is an important component of foods across the globe, especially from East Asia.

tomatillo   A small, round fruit with a distinctive spicy flavor. Tomatillos are a traditional component of many south-of-the-border dishes. To use, remove the papery outer skin, rinse off any sticky residue, and chop like a tomato.

vinegar   An acidic liquid widely used as dressing and seasoning. Many cuisines use vinegars made from different source materials such as fermented grapes, apples, and rice. *See also* balsamic vinegar; cider vinegar; rice vinegar; white vinegar; wine vinegar.

whisk   To rapidly mix, introducing air to the mixture.

Worcestershire sauce   Originally developed in India and containing tamarind, this spicy sauce is used as a seasoning for many meats and other dishes.

zest   Small slivers of peel, usually from a citrus fruit such as lemon, lime, or orange.

zester   A small kitchen tool used to scrape zest off a fruit. A small grater also works well.

Appendix B

Metric Conversion Charts

The scientifically precise calculations needed for baking are not necessary when cooking conventionally or in a slow cooker. This chart is designed for general cooking. If making conversions for baking, grab your calculator and compute the exact figure.

Converting Ounces to Grams

The numbers in the following table are approximate. To reach the exact amount of grams, multiply the number of ounces by 28.35.

Ounces	Grams
1 oz.	30 g
2 oz.	60 g
3 oz.	85 g
4 oz.	115 g
5 oz.	140 g
6 oz.	180 g
7 oz.	200 g
8 oz.	225 g
9 oz.	250 g

continued

Ounces	Grams
10 oz.	285 g
11 oz.	300 g
12 oz.	340 g
13 oz.	370 g
14 oz.	400 g
15 oz.	425 g
16 oz.	450 g

Converting Quarts to Liters

The numbers in the following table are approximate. To reach the exact amount of liters, multiply the number of quarts by 0.95.

Quarts	Liter
1 cup (¼ qt.)	¼ L
1 pint (½ qt.)	½ L
1 qt.	1 L
2 qt.	2 L
2½ qt.	2½ L
3 qt.	2¾ L
4 qt.	3¾ L
5 qt.	4¾ L
6 qt.	5½ L
7 qt.	6½ L
8 qt.	7½ L

Converting Pounds to Grams and Kilograms

The numbers in the following table are approximate. To reach the exact amount of kilograms, multiply the number of pounds by 453.6.

Pounds	Grams; Kilograms
1 lb.	450 g
1½ lb.	675 g
2 lb.	900 g
2½ lb.	1,125 g; 1¼ kg
3 lb.	1,350 g
3½ lb.	1,500 g; 1½ kg
4 lb.	1,800 g
4½ lb.	2k g
5 lb.	2¼ kg
5½ lb.	2½ kg
6 lb.	2¾ kg
6½ lb.	3 kg
7 lb.	3¼ kg
7½ lb.	3½ kg
8 lb.	3¾ kg

Converting Fahrenheit to Celsius

The numbers in the following table are approximate. To reach the exact temperature, subtract 32 from the Fahrenheit reading, multiply the number by 5, then divide by 9.

Fahrenheit	Celsius
170	77
180	82
190	88
200	95
225	110
250	120
300	150
325	165

continues

continued

Fahrenheit	Celsius
350	180
375	190
400	205
425	220
450	230
475	245
500	260

Converting Inches to Centimeters

The numbers in the following table are approximate. To reach the exact number of centimeters, multiply the number of inches by 2.54.

Inches	Centimeters
½ in.	1.5 cm
1 in.	2.5 cm
2 in.	5 cm
3 in.	8 cm
4 in.	10 cm
5 in.	13 cm
6 in.	15 cm
7 in.	18 cm
8 in.	20 cm
9 in.	23 cm
10 in.	25 cm
11 in.	28 cm
12 in.	30 cm

Nutrient Composition of Fruits and Vegetables per 3½ oz. Serving

Food	Protein (g)	Fat (g)	Carb (g)	Calcium (mg)	Phosphorus (mg)	Iron (mg)	Sodium (mg)	Potassium (mg)
Apples	.2	.6	14.5	7	10	.3	1	110
Apricots	1.0	.2	12.8	17	23	.5	1	281
Asparagus	2.5	.2	5	22	62	1.0	2	278
Avocados	2.1	16.4	6.3	10	42	.6	4	604
Bananas	1.1	.2	22.2	8	26	.7	1	370
Beet Greens	2.2	.3	4.6	119	40	3.3	130	570
Beets	1.6	.1	9.9	16	33	.7	60	335
Blackberries	1.2	.9	12.9	32	19	.9	1	170
Blueberries	.7	.5	15.3	15	13	1.0	1	81
Cabbage	1.3	.2	5.4	49	29	.4	20	233
Carrots	1.1	.2	9.7	37	36	.7	47	341
Cauliflower	2.7	.2	5.2	25	56	1.1	13	295
Celery	.9	.1	3.9	39	28	.3	126	341
Collards	4.8	.8	7.5	250	82	1.5	0	450
Garlic	6.2	.2	30.8	29	202	1.5	19	529
Grapefruit	.5	.1	10.6	16	16	.4	1	135
Grapes	1.3	.1	15.7	16	12	.4	3	158
Guava	.8	.6	15	23	42	.9	4	289
Kale	6	8	9	249	93	2.7	75	378

Food	Protein (g)	Fat (g)	Carb (g)	Calcium (g)	Phosphorus (mg)	(mg)	Iron (mg)	Sodium (mg)	Potassium (mg)
Lemons	1.1	.3	8.2	26	16	.6	2	138
Lettuce	1.2	.2	2.5	35	26	2	9	264
Limes	.7	.2	10.5	33	18	.6	2	102
Onions	1.5	.1	8.7	27	36	.5	10	157
Oranges	1	.2	12.2	41	20	.4	1	200
Papaya	.6	1	10	20	16	.3	3	234
Parsley	3.6	.6	8.5	203	63	6.2	45	727
Parsnips	1.7	.5	17.5	50	77	.7	12	541
Peaches	.6	.1	9.7	9	19	.5	1	202
Pears	.7	.4	15.3	8	11	.3	2	130
Peas	6.3	.4	14.4	26	116	1.9	2	316
Peppers, bell	1.2	.2	4.8	9	22	.7	13	213
Peppers, chili	3.7	2.3	18.1	29	78	1.2	0	0
Pineapples	.4	.2	13.7	17	8	.5	1	146
Plums	.5	.1	17.8	18	17	.5	2	299
Pomegranates	.5	.3	16.4	3	8	.3	3	259
Rhubarb	.6	.1	3.7	96	18	.8	2	251

continues

continued

Food	Protein (g)	Fat (g)	Carb (g)	Calcium (g)	Phosphorus (mg)	(mg)	Iron (mg)	Sodium (mg)	Potassium (mg)
Scallions	1.5	.2	8.2	51	39	1	5	231
Spinach	3.2	.3	4.3	93	51	3.1	71	470
Strawberries	.7	.5	8.4	21	21	1	1	164
Tomatoes	1.1	.2	4.7	13	27	.5	3	244
Turnips	1	.2	6.6	39	30	.5	49	268
Watermelons	.5	.2	6.4	7	10	.5	1	100
Yams	1.7	.4	26.3	32	47	.7	10	243

Source: Composition of Foods Handbook #8. U.S. Dept. of Agriculture

Index

M

Q–R

U-V

Check Out These
Best-Sellers

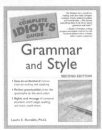
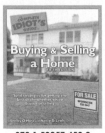
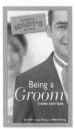
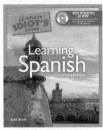
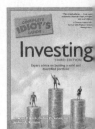
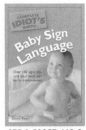
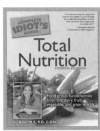
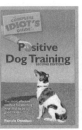
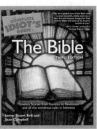
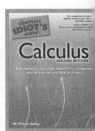
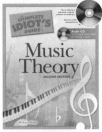
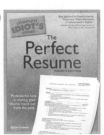
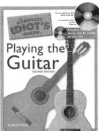
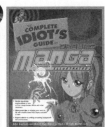
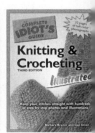